RADIATION ACCIDENTS AND EMERGENCIES IN MEDICINE, RESEARCH, AND INDUSTRY

RADIATION ACCIDENTS AND EMERGENCIES IN MEDICINE, RESEARCH, AND INDUSTRY

Edited by

LAWRENCE H. LANZL, Ph.D.

Department of Radiology and
Argonne Cancer Research Hospital
The University of Chicago
Chicago, Illinois

JOHN H. PINGEL, M.P.H.

Industrial Hygiene and Safety Division
Argonne National Laboratory
Argonne, Illinois

JOHN H. RUST, Ph.D.

Section of Nuclear Medicine
Department of Pharmacology
The University of Chicago
Chicago, Illinois

CHARLES C THOMAS • PUBLISHER

Springfield • Illinois • U.S.A.

Published and Distributed Throughout the World by

CHARLES C THOMAS • PUBLISHER

BANNERSTONE HOUSE

301-327 East Lawrence Avenue, Springfield, Illinois, U.S.A.

NATCHEZ PLANTATION HOUSE

735 North Atlantic Boulevard, Fort Lauderdale, Florida, U.S.A.

Library of Congress Catalog Card Number: 65-11310

With THOMAS BOOKS careful attention is given to all details of manufacturing and design. It is the Publisher's desire to present books that are satisfactory as to their physical qualities and artistic possibilities and appropriate for their particular use. THOMAS BOOKS will be true to those laws of quality that assure a good name and good will.

Printed in the United States of America

H-2

CONTRIBUTORS

RICHARD H. BURR, M.B.A.
Assistant Manager,
Health and Safety Department, Uranium Division
Mallinckrodt Chemical Works
St. Charles, Missouri

WILLIAM R. BUSH, B.A.Sc.
Section Head, Radiation and Industrial Safety Branch
Atomic Energy of Canada Limited
Chalk River, Ontario, Canada

ROBERT J. CATLIN, A.B., C.H.P.
Chief, Health Physics Standards Branch
Division of Licensing and Regulation
U.S. Atomic Energy Commission
Washington, D.C.

THEODORE FIELDS, M.S., C.H.P.
President, Health Physics Associates
Highland Park, Illinois

HOWARD R. FISH, JR., B.S.E.E.
Assistant Electrical Engineer
Industrial Hygiene and Safety Division
Argonne National Laboratory
Argonne, Illinois

EDWARD H. FORGOTSON, M.D., L.L.M.
Deputy Special Assistant to the President for Mental Retardation
The White House
Washington, D.C.

ROBERT G. GALLAGHAR, A.B., C.H.P.
President, Applied Health Physics, Inc.
Bethel Park, Pennsylvania

LEE GEMMELL, M.S., C.H.P.
Associate Head, Health Physics Division
Brookhaven National Laboratory
Upton, L.I., New York

LEON O. JACOBSON, M.D.
Director, Argonne Cancer Research Hospital, and
Chairman, Department of Medicine,
The University of Chicago
Chicago, Illinois

WILLIAM S. JOHNSON, SR., M.S., C.H.P.
Regional Manager
Eberline Instrument Corporation
Danville, California

ROBERT S. KLECKNER, A.B.
Science Writer
Chicago Sun Times
Chicago, Illinois

ROBERT S. LANDAUER, SR., Ph.D., C.H.P.
Physicist, Radiation Center
Cook County Hospital
Chicago, Illinois

LAWRENCE H. LANZL, Ph.D., C.H.P.
Associate Professor of Medical Physics
Argonne Cancer Research Hospital, and
Department of Radiology
The University of Chicago
Chicago, Illinois

GEORGE V. LeROY, M.D.
Professor, Department of Medicine
The University of Chicago
Chicago, Illinois

JOSEPH C. MALONEY, B.E.
Chief, Decontamination Branch
U.S. Army Nuclear Defense Laboratory
Edgewood Arsenal, Maryland

MONT G. MASON
Manager, Medicine, Health and Safety
Uranium Division
Mallinckrodt Chemical Works
St. Charles, Missouri

RAYMOND T. MOORE, M.D.
Program Director, Radiological Health
U.S. Public Health Service
Department of Health, Education and Welfare
Region VII—Dallas, Texas

RICHARD B. O'BRIEN, B.S.
Supervisor, Health Physics and Safety
General Electric Company
Nuclear Materials and Propulsion Operation
Idaho Falls, Idaho

DONALD OKEN, M.D.
Associate Director, Psychosomatic and
Psychiatric Institute
Michael Reese Hospital
Chicago, Illinois

CLAIRE C. PALMITER, B.S.
U.S. Atomic Energy Commission Representative
Secretariat of Federal Radiation Council
Executive Office Building
Washington, D.C.

JOHN H. PINGEL, M.P.H., C.H.P.
Health Physicist, Industrial Hygiene and Safety Division
Argonne National Laboratory
Argonne, Illinois

JOHN H. RUST, D.V.M., Ph.D., D.Sc.
Professor and Head, Section of Nuclear
Medicine, Department of Pharmacology
The University of Chicago
Chicago, Illinois

JACOB SEDLET, Ph.D.
Chemist, Industrial Hygiene and Safety Division
Argonne National Laboratory
Argonne, Illinois

LYLE D. THOMAS, M.S.
Associate Regional Program Director
Division of Radiological Health
U.S. Public Health Service
Department of Health, Education and Welfare
Chicago, Illinois

CARL M. UNRUH, M.S., C.H.P.
Manager, Radiological Development and Calibrations
Radiation Protection Operation
Hanford Laboratories
General Electric Company
Richland, Washington

EDWARD J. VALLARIO, B.S.
Health Physicist
Division of Operational Safety
U.S. Atomic Energy Commission
Washington, D.C.

GEORGE L. VOELZ, M.D.
Assistant Director for Health Services
Health and Safety Division
U.S. Atomic Energy Commission
Idaho Operations Office
Idaho Falls, Idaho

MILO D. VOSS, B.S., C.H.P.
Associate Physicist and Group Leader
Radiological Services Group
Ames Laboratory, U.S. Atomic Energy Commission, and
Iowa State University of Science and Technology
Ames, Iowa

G. HOYT WHIPPLE, Ph.D., C.H.P.
Professor of Radiological Health and
Radiological Safety Officer
School of Public Health
University of Michigan
Ann Arbor, Michigan

PAUL L. ZIEMER, Ph.D.
Assistant Professor of Health Physics
Department of Bionucleonics
Purdue University
Lafayette, Indiana

F. RAYMOND ZINTZ
Radiological Assistance Coordinator
Division of Operational Safety
U.S. Atomic Energy Commission
Washington, D.C.

PREFACE

THIS VOLUME constitutes the proceedings of the *Symposium on Radiation Accidents and Emergencies in Medicine, Research, and Industry* which was held in Chicago on December 19 and 20, 1963. The symposium was initiated by the Midwest Chapter of the Health Physics Society. The Chapter was later joined in its sponsorship by the Radiation and Medical Physics Society of Illinois and the Chicago Section of the American Industrial Hygiene Association.

The persons who attended the symposium came from a variety of geographical locations. These included twenty-eight continental states, Hawaii, Puerto Rico, Canada, and Austria. The percentage institutional representation of the attendees was 28 per cent industrial or commercial, 17 per cent U.S. Atomic Energy Commission or its contractors, 14 per cent public health, 12 per cent space and defense, 11 per cent university, and 7 per cent hospital. The remainder included persons from insurance companies, labor unions, and research institutions, as well as private individuals.

The success of a symposium depends on the work of many persons. The operating committees were composed of the following persons: General Chairman, Robert V. Wheeler; Arrangements, Carroll D. Hampleman; Finance and Registration, Robert K. Clark; Printing and Advertising, Albert G. Januska; Publicity, Stanley R. Lasuk; and Program and Publications, John H. Pingel, Chairman, Enrico F. Conti, Lawrence H. Lanzl, and William B. Rivkin.

During the symposium, the following persons served as Session Chairmen: Robert K. Clark, Enrico F. Conti, Donald M. Gardiner, Lawrence H. Lanzl, Walter S. Moos, John R. Novak, C. Maurice Patterson, and William B. Rivkin.

The symposium was supported in part by the Division of Radiological Health, U.S. Department of Health, Education and Welfare. The encouragement and interest of James G. Terrill, Jr., and Raymond T. Moore of the Division is gratefully acknowledged.

The publication of these proceedings has been supported in part by a grant from the Rockefeller Foundation to the Section of Nuclear Medicine, Department of Pharmacology, The University of Chicago. The Editors wish further to express their thanks to Dolores M. Trefelner for typing the manuscript and to Elisabeth F. Lanzl for many valuable suggestions in manuscript preparation as well as indexing.

L. H. L.
J. H. P.
J. H. R.

CONTENTS

RADIATION ACCIDENTS AND EMERGENCIES IN MEDICINE, RESEARCH, AND INDUSTRY

INTRODUCTION

SCOPE OF THE PROBLEM

LAWRENCE H. LANZL

Department of Radiology and
Argonne Cancer Research Hospital
The University of Chicago
Chicago, Illinois

THE POSSIBILITY that a radiation accident or emergency may occur is the concern of every serious person involved in the use of ionizing radiations. Such a person may be, for example, a research physcisist, biologist, chemist, a practicing physician, reactor engineer, public health or safety officer, member of the armed forces, administrator, or especially a health physicist. The symposium, whose proceedings comprise this volume, was organized in an attempt to cover most of the pertinent aspects of pure emergency and accident situations from a broad point of view.

In this volume, papers dealing with related subjects are grouped under chapter headings. The discussions which followed presentation of the papers are recorded either directly after a given paper or following a group of papers.

The program for the symposium was planned according to topics rather than in a case study format, although a detailed examination of different accident situations could be an effective way of presenting the subject. The classification of radiations or radioactive materials involved in accidents is covered in Unruh's paper in the first chapter. This is followed by a paper expressing the views of Kleckner on the publicity of radiation accidents. His comments can be regarded as typical of members of an open and concerned society.

Immediately after an accident, certain actions (Voss) including screening (Pingel) and possibly bioassaying (Sedlet) need to be initiated. These actions pose problems, by virtue of the nature of radiation, which do not exist in any other types of accidents and emergencies. The anxieties of individuals and groups, and other psychological problems which arise in emergency situations, are discussed by Oken. These topics constitute the second chapter.

The present status of medical science with respect to reduction of the internal contamination of victims is thoroughly surveyed by Voelz in the third chapter, together with the problem of maximum permissible levels of internal contamination (LeRoy). Most hospitals are not equipped to handle readioactively contaminated individuals. Landauer, who has made a study of hospitals in Illinois to determine how this deficiency may be overcome, presents his views here. In addition, this chapter contains methods of external decontamination of uninjured personnel (Burr and Mason).

The art and the science of decontaminating equipment and materials have been vigorously pursued during the last two decades. In Chapter 4, Gemmell reviews both old and new techniques; Bush surveys world-wide existing standards for permissible radioactivity levels on surfaces following decontamination. The problem of large-scale outdoor decontamination under cold-weather and winter conditions has been reported on for the first time in open literature (Maloney). Disposal of contaminated waste in the SL-1 (Stationary Low Power Plant) reactor accident in Idaho led, to some extent, to the abandoning of the concept that only centralized, established waste disposal sites should be used (O'Brien).

Chapter 5 covers some specific problems, such as those posed by radium contamination (Fields; see also Gallaghar), which the radiologist or gynecologist often faces. On a larger scale, the vast alpha-particle emitter contamination problem which results when a non-nuclear explosion (chemical part) of an atomic weapon takes place is the subject of Johnson's paper. His measurements are the most extensive ever made in this field. Specifications for instruments required in accident situations (Fish) and emergency dose criteria (Vallario and Catlin) are included here.

Administrative aspects are considered in Chapter 6. Forgotson discusses legal liability problems encountered in accident situations. Gallaghar, who represents a private firm dealing with radiation incidents, covers reporting and documentation of emergencies. The unusual position of universities poses special problems in emergency planning (Ziemer). Management problems such as emergency policy, training, and drills are discussed by Whipple.

In Chapter 7, four representatives of agencies of the federal government explain the far-reaching government services and regulations, including the radiological teams of the several agencies which give prompt and generous assistance in case of a radiation accident or emergency.

The final chapter constitutes a departure from the practical problems of dealing with radiation incidents. It is concerned instead with the moral aspects and their implications for society.

Dr. Leon O. Jacobson, in his remarks at the opening of the symposium, highlighted some of the scientific events, and their discoverers, of the last twenty years. Dr. Jacobson himself was one of the first life-science workers to take part in the Nation's nuclear energy program.

Explanation of Terms

It is appropriate to include explanations of some of the more important terms used in the following papers. The usual definition of an accident as an event that takes place without one's expectation is generally a valid one for a *radiation accident* provided, of course, that radiation is somehow implicated. This definition may seem incongruent with the often-heard remark, "Accidents will happen," which implies that they are to be expected. Thus, to be semantically more correct, we might say that an accident is an event that may take place at an unexpected time, and possibly in an unexpected place.

The word *incident* is widely used among radiation protection workers. It refers to all accidents, and to those other similar events which are expected to result occasionally in undesirable release of radioactive materials.

The term *radiation emergency* is used in two different senses: the more conventional meaning suggests an unforseen combination of circumstances involving radiation, which calls for immediate action. However, the report of the National Committee on Radiation Protection and Measurements states (1) that "A radiation emergency is an accident, or other event out of the ordinary, that threatens to expose people to more than 25 r in one week." This latter definition is not widely used at the present time, but may become so in the future.

The unit of exposure, the *roentgen,* and the unit of absorbed dose, the *rad,* are well known (1, 2, 3), and their definitions do not need to be further elaborated upon. On the other hand, the term *rem* has undergone many changes of definition in recent years. The letters of the unit were associated for many years with their original derivation from the initials of the words "roentgen equivalent man." In the 1961 report of the National Committee on Radiation Protection and Measurement, *Handbook 76* (2), the rem was defined as the dose unit of the *relative biological effectiveness (RBE).* RBE is used to compare the effectiveness of absorbed radiation delivered in different ways. The 1956 and 1959 Reports of the International Commission on Radiological Units and Measurements (3, 4), however, did not *define* RBE and its unit, the rem, but categorized them as "recognized symbols." Here, the RBE was stated to be numerically equal to the product of the dose in rads and an agreed conventional value of the RBE in terms of the effect of a particular form of radiation. Thus, both the National Committee and the International Commission now relate the rem to absorbed dose rather than to exposure.

For purposes of regulatory control of exposure of individuals to radiation, the definition of the rem is, in one sense, simplified in comparison with the strict scientific definitions referred to above. Even though this simplification does tend to lead to confusion at times, it is justified for health protection purposes. The regulatory definition is published in the Code of Federal Regulations (5). It states: "The rem is a measure of the dose of any ionizing radiation to body tissue in terms of its estimated biological effect relative to a dose of one roentgen (r) of x-rays. . . . For the purpose of the regulations in this part, any of the following is considered to be equivalent to a dose of one rem:

"1.) *A dose of 1r due to x- or gamma radiation,*
"2.) *A dose of 1 rad due to x-, gamma,* or beta radiation,
"3.) A dose of 0.1 rad due to neutrons or high energy protons,
"4.) A dose of 0.05 rad due to particles heavier than protons and with sufficient energy to reach the lens of the eye. . . ."

The rem thus is considered to be equivalent simultaneously to both the exposure and the absorbed dose, which is approximately true for muscle and bone at, say, 400 kvp x-rays, and for muscle at 100 kvp x-rays; however, it differs by a factor of three in skeletal bone for 100 kvp x-rays.

The unit of radioactivity, the *curie*, has been defined, for a number of years, as 3.7×10^{10} disintegrations per second (except for radium). For regulatory purposes, a special definition for natural uranium (and similarly thorium) has been added (5), namely, ". . . one curie of natural uranium means the sum of 3.7×10^{10} disintegrations per second from uranium-238 plus 3.7×10^{10} disintegrations per second from uranium-234 plus 9×10^{8} disintegrations per second from uranium-235."

The word *"contamination"* is frequently used in many of the papers. Its meaning in this volume refers strictly to the presence of radioactive substances. In health physics parlance, the terms "alpha contamination" and "beta contamination" are common, and refer to the contaminant from which alpha particles or beta particles are emitted. The correct terminology, therefore, is *"alpha particle emitter* or *alpha-emitting contamination"* and *"beta particle emitter* or *beta-emitting contamination,"* and this terminology is used throughout these papers.

Where other special terms are used, an effort has been made to define them in the papers in which they occur. The index will be of help in locating these definitions.

REFERENCES

1. *Exposure to Radiation in an Emergency.* National Committee on Radiation Protection and Measurements. Report No. 29, Section of Nuclear Medicine, The University of Chicago, p. 8, January 1962.
2. NBS Handbook 76, *Medical X-ray Protection up to Three Million Volts.* Recommendations of the National Committee on Radiation Protection and Measurements, NCRP Report No. 26, U.S. Government Printing Office, Washington, D.C., 1961.
3. NBS Handbook 62, *Report of the International Commission on Radiological Units and Measurements (ICRU) 1956.* U.S. Government Printing Office, Washington, D.C., 1957.

4. NBS Handbook 78, *Report of the International Commission on Radiological Units and Measurements (ICRU) 1959.* U.S. Government Printing Office, Washington, D.C., 1961.
5. Code of Federal Regulations, Title 10, Atomic Energy; Part 20, Standards for Protection Again Radiation. *Federal Register,* U.S. Government Printing Office, Washington, D.C., November 17, 1960.

STRIDES OF THE PAST AND PRESENT

LEON O. JACOBSON*

Department of Medicine and
Argonne Cancer Research Hospital
The University of Chicago
Chicago, Illinois

THE PAST 25 years have seen a great expansion of personnel in the field of radiation physics. In 1940, it would have been possible to count the health physicists without any difficulty: today virtually hundreds are engaged in such research, as is witnessed by the present symposium on radiation accidents and emergencies. It gives me great pleasure to pay tribute to some of the pioneers:

Dr. Robert S. Landauer (see page 122) has contributed through his teaching of radiation physics to radiologists over several decades and through his personal surveillance of the radiation installations of numerous hospitals here in the midwestern part of the country. More recently, he has served on various commissions advising the State of Illinois legislature on radiation control. The late Dr. Gioacchino Failla established the first laboratory for hospital radiation physics in the United States some forty years ago, and continued throughout his life to improve the knowledge and understanding of the process of radiation absorption. His experimental work is a monument of precision and completeness. Herbert M. Parker, the physicist who, with the English radiologist Ralston Paterson, initiated rules (now known as the Paterson-Parker Rules) for radium implantation, was closely associated with the Metallurgical Laboratory of the Manhattan Project.

Dr. Russell Morgan, also formerly of the Metallurgical Laboratory,

---

*Dr. Jacobson has pioneered in work on the protection of the hematopoietic system from the deleterious effects of radiations, including the role of the spleen in preventing and repairing damage. He was given the Borden Award for his work on the mechanism of blood formation and control.

has contributed greatly in recent years toward the reduction of dose to patients and hospital personnel through the application of image intensifiers for remote viewing. Dr. John E. Rose, who designed many of the nation's hospital radium plants, has been a pioneer in the development of dosimeters used in health protection work. The physicist, Leonidas Marinelli, has been responsible for careful experimental work on measuring radiation output of isotopes, and on the effects of radiation on bone, and, perhaps more relevant to the subject at hand, on the re-enactment of a reactor accident and the dose evaluation of persons who were unfortunately too close to a run-away reactor. Outstanding physicians, including Robert S. Stone, the late Dr. Simeon Cantril and Dr. Henry A. Blair, have shown great interest in the area of health physics. During World War II, Dr. Stone pioneered the use of neutrons for therapy. Later in the war, these three medical scientists did much to inform atomic energy workers about the dangers of radiation and to extend knowledge of those dangers by careful experimentation.

At the beginning of 1940, when I first became associated with this work, I was quite unaware of the remarkable progress already made by a number of individuals. It was a great experience to see the team of physicists and biologists working together to establish a basis for devising protective measures against the biological effects of radiation. Here we should not forget the work of Dr. Jacob Furth who, as early as the 1930's, had already done some magnificent work on the chronic effects of low-dose radiation delivered over an extended period of time. His studies served in part as a basis for the permissible levels which were being used at the beginning of World War II. The late physicist, Dr. Egon Lorenz in Bethesda, Maryland, also did outstanding work in the same area of extended low-dose irradiation.

It is also important to remember that the great industries of this country had long recognized the necessity for a sound program in industrial medicine, and had expended a great deal of effort and time in educating their workers and the general populace in the need for advanced methods of protection in this era of greatly increased work with radioactive materials.

The benefits derived from the collaboration of specialists in many fields is typified by an incident that occurred here during World

War II, and I am sure that many similar experiences could be cited. The Manhattan District Metallurgical Laboratory, Oak Ridge Laboratory, and the Hanford Works Plant were, of necessity, protected by great secrecy. I would venture to guess that, on the campus of the University of Chicago, even at the time of the pilot operation of the first nuclear reactor, not a single individual outside the project knew what was going on in the stands below Stagg Field. One day, a man appeared in the Dermatology Section of the University Clinics complaining of a skin eruption on his hands. The late Dr. Stephen Rothman, who was then head of Dermatology, said, after looking him over carefully, "Have you had exposure to radiation?" The man replied, "Oh, yes. I've been carrying it around in large chunks for weeks." So, Dr. Rothman naturally put down as a diagnosis, "radiation dermatitis." We cleared* Dr. Rothman the following week.

Research on experimental animals, efforts by Government agencies to determine the dispersal and persistence of radioactive particles from atomic explosions, the concern of international authorities for the exposure of doctors, nurses and patients to therapeutic and diagnostic irradiation, all indicate that we do not as yet know with any certainty what the lower limits for radiation should be for strontium-90, for example, or even for diagnostic x-rays. The continued cooperation between the biologists and physicists is our hope for the solution of these problems.

On the other hand, a number of interesting studies suggests that radiation injury can be prevented and, to some extent, can be treated. In this connection, the work of Dr. Harvey Patt, at the Argonne National Laboratory, and Dr. Eugene P. Cronkite, at the Brookhaven National Laboratory, may be mentioned. These men have shown, in a piece of work that has not yet been properly recognized, and which I consider one of the most important discoveries of the last twenty years, that it is possible to decrease the effect of radiation by a factor of two. Again, Dr. F. H. Gardner and Dr. J. H. Lawrence showed as early as 1938 that the administration of estrogens to rats ten days before irradiation increased the LD_{50} by a factor of two. I have

*Federal Bureau of Investigation report followed by security clearance—an investigation of a person's character and background to determine trustworthiness, and indoctrination concerning the possession of secret or secret-related knowledge.

mentioned these discoveries not only because they are important, but also because they indicate what remains to be done. It seems fantastic that, after at least twenty-five years, we do not know yet why estrogens will protect. In fact, it is not known with certainty why any substance protects.

As far as my own work on radioprotection is concerned, it was really by chance that I discovered that one could give an animal a lethal dose of radiation and then keep it alive with transplanted blood-forming tissue. While there is no doubt that this can be done, not only in animals, but also in human beings, this is not a practical method of protection from ionizing radiation in the human; nor is it yet practical to give pre-medication for protection.

Both pre-medication and post-medication are areas in which the biologist will need the help of the radiation physicist in order to be successful. I must emphasize that, in my opinion, prophylaxis is a most important aspect—and this is the job of the health physicist. I hope you can successfully carry us to the point where we no longer have radiation injuries or accidents and, God willing, no more bombs.

Chapter I

ACCIDENTS INVOLVING RADIATION OR RADIOACTIVE MATERIALS

RADIATION EMERGENCIES: TYPES AND MECHANISMS

CARL M. UNRUH*

Radiation Protection Operation
Hanford Laboratories
General Electric Company
Richland, Washington

ANYONE WORKING with radioactive materials may have a radiation accident. This should be recognized as a basic fact requiring consideration and emergency action planning by all who work with radioactive materials. Such accidents can occur in spite of all the care, design, and engineering considerations that may be included in the construction and use of a facility whether it is large or small.

The course of events in any radiation emergency may be divided into four phases: Occurrence, Emergency, Recovery, and Restoration.

Occurrence Phase. The occurrence phase encompasses the happenings immediately preceding the radiation accident and includes the physical event itself, the sounding of any automatically activated alarms or warning signals that may be provided, and the immediate evacuation of the facility, if necessary.

Emergency Phase. The emergency phase encompasses all action which may be taken promptly to save lives and to protect property. To be effective, these actions will be taken by personnel in the immediate vicinity at the time of the event. Only equipment and resources immediately available will be of value in this phase.

Recovery Phase. There is no sharp line of distinction between

*Work performed under Contract No. AT(45-1)-1350 for the U.S. Atomic Energy Commission.

the emergency and the recovery phase. In the latter, actions are planned, organized, and directed toward recovery from the results of the event. Additional equipment and personnel may be brought into action during the recovery phase, and consultation services may be obtained. The recovery phase results in the establishment of control over the situation.

Restoration Phase. This phase encompasses the program for restoring conditions to their original state, establishing some intermediate state of acceptability, or abandoning the restoration efforts.

As a basis for beginning our discussion, we should review the definitions of three simple words which will be used throughout the symposium. First, "accident"—an accident is defined as an event that takes place without foresight or expectation. Second, "emergency"—an emergency is an unforeseen combination of circumstances which calls for immediate action. Third, "plan"—a plan is a method of action or procedure. The key to success in meeting a radiation emergency is to have plans as well as resources of equipment and trained personnel available in an adequate state of readiness so that the necessary immediate action can be taken. Very commonly, immediate action can prevent a radiation emergency from spreading and enlarging and can thus effectively control the consequences of the emergency.

In the discussion of the types and mechanisms of radiation emergencies, three major groups may be considered, namely: 1) the nature of the source of radiation, 2) the mechanisms of loss of radiation source control, and 3) the consequences of loss of radiation source control.

I. Nature of the Source of Radiation

Radiation sources used by medical, research, and industrial facilities may be broadly classified as radiation generating machines, unsealed radiation sources, and sealed radiation sources. The use of radiation-generating machines leads to the simplest control actions. Most commonly, the use of these machines can only result in external radiation exposure problems. With unsealed radiation sources, the potential for external radiation exposure, internal deposition of radioactive material in the body, and the general spread of radioactive contamination exists. In the use of sealed radiation sources, the primary potential hazard is the external radiation exposure of personnel.

In the care required and the hazards involved in handling any radioactive source, the physical and biological properties of the radioactive source material are important considerations. For example, high-energy gamma-ray sources require extensive shielding, while low-energy gamma-ray sources or alpha- and beta-ray emitting sources are easily shielded. The biological factors involved in human ingestion of various radioactive materials play an important part in determining the degree of care required and the protection program necessary for the safe handling of unsealed radioactive materials. Clearly, the biologically hazardous materials dictate more rigorous equipment design and reliability, and more detailed procedures to assure their containment, than do materials which are not biologically hazardous.

Radiation-Generating Machines. X-ray machines and particle accelerators are commonly used radiation-generating machines. They are distinguished from other radiation sources in that they may be switched on or off at will; also, no source storage problems are encountered. In the use of neutron-generating machines, care should be taken to assure that the neutrons do not activate the target or nearby materials to create a radioactive source which will not be "shut off" when the machine is shut off. Radiation contamination problems are not usually encountered in the operation of x-ray generating equipment. Care should be taken to assure that the operation of all radiation-generating machines is limited to authorized personnel under authorized conditions.

Unsealed Radiation Sources. Unsealed radioactive materials are another source of radiation encountered in medical, research, and industrial facilities. Emergencies resulting from the loss of control of radioactive contaminants from unsealed radiation sources generally differ from accidents with sealed sources or x-rays in that there is a potential likelihood for extensive contamination of property, and that the mode of exposure of involved individuals is more complex. The spread of radioactive materials from an unsealed source to personnel, equipment and the environs can create exposure, contamination, and internal deposition problems.

Unsealed radioactive materials are handled in hoods, glove boxes, or shielded cells. Control of these materials is maintained by providing a positive barrier between the operation facilities and the processing area, adequate shielding, and proper air flow patterns. Ideally, unsealed sources thus confined may be regarded as expanded versions of the normally handled sealed sources of radioactive materials. Handling problems are considerably more difficult, however, because the total amount of material is usually greater, and because there are much greater chances for containment breakdown due to the penetrations through the source containment barrier which are necessary for conducting the programmed work.

Sealed Radiation Sources. A very commonly used source of radiation is the sealed source. A sealed radiation source is usually small in size physically, namely, less than an inch or two in its maximum dimension. The radioactive material is firmly contained within the source capsule to prevent the spread of contamination. Sources of this type may emit gamma, neutron, beta, or alpha radiations separately or in combinations, depending upon the radioisotope contained and the design of the source capsule. For sealed radiation sources emitting alpha or beta radiation, a thin window is necessary to permit the emergence of a useful fraction of the emitted particles from the source container. With thin-window sources, care in handling is a vital consideration to prevent window rupture. Sealed sources emit radiation continuously and therefore generally require some degree of shielding and isolation from personnel when not in use.

Radiation accidents with fixed or sealed sources such as x-ray machines and cobalt-60 irradiation units are often due to an uncontrolled approach of persons to the radiation source. This can be the result of uncontrolled movement of the source, or of uncontrolled movement of persons in the vicinity of the source.

II. Mechanisms of Loss of Radiation Source Control

The mechanisms of loss of control over radioactive materials are a function of the type of source material being handled, as well as of the design of the facility where the source is being used. All radioactive sources and radiation-generating equipment may be managed by means of control of personnel and control of radioactive materials.

A breakdown in either of these may lead to a radiation emergency. With the exception of a nuclear excursion or criticality event, the mechanisms causing a radiation emergency are frequently identical to those in more conventional emergencies. Accidents in which the spill of noxious materials, fire, explosions, vehicular accidents, and equipment failures occur can lead to serious radiation emergencies if radioactive materials are involved. Radiation design engineers attempt to build into the facilities a degree of protection dependent upon the consequences of possible radiation emergencies.

For the handling of extremely hazardous radioactive materials, a double-containment principle which provides two independent barriers between operating personnel and radioactive materials may be appropriate. Additionally, electronic instrumentation for promptly indicating any loss of control may be included as a fundamental part of a radiation facility.

Control of Personnel. Control of personnel is usually accomplished by posting radiation signs and erecting barriers. Accidents involving personnel may occur whenever an unauthorized entry into a processing area occurs. A particularly important factor in assuring control of personnel is the appropriate and frequently reviewed use of a good training program stressing the importance of rigid compliance with safe handling procedures for all radioactive materials, and the observance of all posted radiation protection regulations. Thorough training has repeatedly yielded good dividends in radiation emergency prevention. Its fundamental importance for the prevention of radiation emergencies due to personnel cannot be overstressed.

Control of Radiation-Generating Machines. The control of radiation-generating equipment is accomplished by providing for authorized operation after thorough inspection of the areas to be irradiated. Radiation-generating equipment and the irradiation areas should be designed to prevent unauthorized use. Operation of equipment by persons unauthorized to do so and hence not fully aware of the precautions to be taken can create a loss of radiation control. Equipment locks and safety devices should be installed to prevent this.

Due to poor training or violation of operating procedures, personnel might remain within the irradiation area during equipment operation, resulting in their unplanned exposure. The use of an appropriate radiation alarm system to signal the presence of radiation can provide substantial protection against such occurrences. Such a system prevents accidents due to a situation in which radiation-generating equipment may be turned on without the knowledge of those operating the equipment.

Conventional accidents such as fire, explosions, power failures, vehicular accidents, etc., will not generally result in any loss of control of radiation-generating equipment.

Control of Unsealed Radiation Sources. Radioactive materials should be appropriately contained and shielded at all times. Strict control of radioactive materials in the form of unsealed sources is necessary to prevent the contamination of plant facilities and personnel. Serious radiation emergencies can lead to a general spread of contamination to the environs and to a large number of people who may be totally unaware of this occurrence. Only authorized, well-trained personnel should be permitted to handle and work with unsealed radiation sources.

Although unsealed sources are considered to be uncontained, they are, in fact, contained within hoods, glove boxes, cells, or similar enclosures. Breaks in these containers can provide a leakage path resulting in the general spread of radioactive contamination.

The possibility of accidental spill is high during the transfer of unsealed radioactive materials such as liquids or powders. Transfer mechanisms and equipment should be designed in as "fail-safe" a manner as possible. Various equipment failures may occur as the result of errors in processing steps. Such errors can rapidly lead to radiation emergencies through fires, explosions, and general loss of control of the materials.

With the exception of a violent explosion or major fire involving radioactive materials, one may anticipate that the general loss of control in a building will not immediately contaminate the plant environs. Prompt action to regain control of the situation can limit the contamination to the personnel and equipment directly involved.

In locations where large quantities of fissionable materials are being processed, rigid criticality controls are also necessary. These should prevent the assembly of a critical mass of material. The consequences of a criticality event are generally well known. They may result in excessive radiation exposure, damage to equipment and plant facilities, and a general spread of radioactive materials. Experience has proven that prompt evacuation of personnel following the detection of a criticality event can indeed be a life-saving operation. If the inventory contains critical masses of fissionable material, criticality alarms should be provided throughout the facility to give an immediate evacuation signal to all personnel.

Control of Sealed Radiation Sources. Many accidents occur when radioactive source materials are not properly stored upon completion of their use. Poor source storage practices and inadequate training of personnel may result in unauthorized use of sealed source materials which can lead to source rupture and excessive personnel exposure.

Occasionally, poor housekeeping and inadequate operator training can result in physical loss of a radiation source. Loss can also be due to equipment failure, or negligence on the part of the equipment operator. For example, the source in an isotope irradiation unit may become detached from its retracting cable, so that the mere winding of the cable back to the storage position is not sufficient to guarantee the shielding of the source. Actual radiation measurements should be made when using radiation sources to assure that they are properly secured, before an area is released to general personnel occupancy.

With poor handling practices, the sealed-source container may be crushed by a piece of equipment or ruptured in dropping. Source ruptures are hazardous in that an unsealed source is created in a facility or area designed for sealed sources only. If contamination control is not adequately handled immediately following source rupture, general contamination of the immediate area results.

Continued use of a sealed source in chemically corrosive atmospheres may damage the source container. Sources used in corrosive atmospheres should be examined frequently to assure container integrity. An even better course of action is to use containers resistant to such atmospheres.

If improperly prepared, many sealed sources may tend to build up internal gas pressures. Certain sources have been known to swell and eventually rupture due to internal pressure alone. Source manufacturers attempt to guard against this difficulty; however, each user of sealed sources must make routine inspections for signs of the buildup of internal pressure.

Fires, explosions, and other types of conventional accidents which may occur in the vicinity of locations where sealed sources are used can rupture or displace such sources, leading to a possible radiation emergency.

III. Consequences of Loss of Radiation Source Control

The extent of involvement in terms of severity and type of radiation exposure, types and number of people exposed, interaction with the public domain, and the duration of the radiation emergency, is a function of the source of radiation and of the mechanism of the accident. Each possible course of an accident requires careful examination to assure that emergency planning and the implementation of emergency plans will be effective and timely.

Radiation-Generating Machines. Loss of control of radiation-generating machines results in an external radiation exposure problem. The radiation field will generally be limited to the facility where the radiation-generating machine is located. No contamination will result, and consequently, no internal deposition with its attendant problems. There is no expense for decontamination of equipment or personnel. Emergency action to terminate the radiation field is accomplished simply by turning off the machine. There is no cost for the cleanup of a radiation emergency of this type.

Unsealed Radiation Sources. Loss of control of unsealed radiation sources leads to the most serious and also most costly radiation emergencies. This loss of control may result in external radiation exposure, internal deposition, contamination of personnel and plant facilities, and the possible spread of radioactive materials to the public domain. The major cost in such a radiation emergency will be for the decontamination of equipment and environs. Decontamination costs depend on the amount of radioactive material in the unsealed sources and the extent of spreading of the contamination. Costs may vary from tens of dollars for decontaminating a simple hood to millions of dollars for cleanups involving very large amounts of radioactive materials. Generally, good radiological design can provide a facility capable of containing the bulk of the contamination, thereby limiting decontamination costs to efforts applied within the facility. Possible internal depositions and external exposures may result in law suits for damage by the exposed individuals. The costs of defending or meeting judgments in these cases vary widely.

Sealed Radiation Sources. Consequences from loss of control of sealed radiation sources in many cases parallel those of radiation-generating machines. As long as the sealed sources remain intact, the radiation emergencies resulting may be classified as external exposure problems. If the source is not lost or removed from the facility, only personnel in the facility at the time will be involved. No decontamination expenses will be incurred. Internal deposition cannot result. If, however, the source container is ruptured or broken in the course of the radiation emergency, a situation paralleling that with unsealed sources will occur. Usually, the total inventory of radioactive materials in sealed sources is low compared to that in unsealed sources. A good standard of practice for minimizing source rupture is to encapsulate each radiation source in a double-walled casing and, if at all possible, to schedule routine inspections of the inner container for possible rupture.

IV. Conclusion

The mechanisms of radiation emergencies generally are identical with those of the more conventional emergencies. Unique to radiation emergencies are the possibilities of external exposure of personnel, internal deposition of radioactive materials within the body, and radioactive contamination of personnel, plant facilities and the public domain.

Radiation emergency planning should consider each mode of loss of control of radiation sources and the consequences of such a loss of control. The radiation emergency planning should detail the necessary actions and indicate where equipment and personnel resources are available. All radiation emergency planning should remain flexible. One should not hesitate to deviate from a previous plan in order to meet the specific needs of a given emergency. Routine training and practice sessions for rescue, radiation protection, and operating personnel should prove invaluable in assuring proper immediate action following any given radiation emergency. The Boy Scouts' motto, "Be Prepared," may be considered as a golden rule for meeting a radiation emergency situation.

PUBLICITY OF RADIATION ACCIDENTS*

ROBERT S. KLECKNER

Science Writer
Chicago Sun-Times
Chicago, Illinois

THE FACT that radiation accidents happen, and the consequences of their happening, are known in the public mind. There are other known facts about radiation: it cannot be sensed, so that persons can be exposed without knowing it; articles which are irradiated can become radioactive; radioactive materials can escape into the public domain. It is also well known that explosions of atomic weapons spread radioactive materials all around the world, and that radiation can produce lethal effects.

The atomic energy installations are exceedingly careful about the handling of radioactive sources. Particularly in the past, places where work with radioactive materials was going on were "off limits" to the public, and the work in general was kept secret. This resulted in poor communication of the true state of affairs to the public. In addition, there was (and usually is) poor communication of the meaning of the language used in discussing radiation hazards.

All this adds up to a fear situation for which all the elements are present. The public knows that it can be harmed by radiation; it is not able to sense or know when this may occur; it has not had assurance of the right sort that it is being properly protected, and it has not always been given the facts.

The scientific community has not always taken the public into its confidence. It should assume a large part of the responsibility for solving this problem of communication. The mass media have not been used to full advantage. They stand ready to help if you can agree as to how they can help.

To some extent, it is the job of the scientists to help educate the

*See also R. G. Gallaghar, p. 239, D. Oken, p. 42f., M. D. Voss, 32, P. L. Ziemer, p. 262.

public through speeches at service and civic groups, before parent-teacher associations, and the like. It is their job to reach the news media in simple and understandable language—in words which a fourth grader can understand. News media, in my opinion, have done a fair job of publicizing what material they get from you and your scientific colleagues. We have to depend on you for accuracy.

When hazards are discussed properly, the public takes things calmly, except perhaps for a screwball fringe. A well-informed public, kept up to date on atomic developments in all their connotations, will not panic about dangers.

In its 1960 report, the Committee on Biological Effects of Atomic Radiation concluded that developments since the 1956 report indicate clearly that radiation in all its forms will play an increasing role in the lives of all mankind. The uses of nuclear fission will continue to expand and potential radiation hazards will increase accordingly. Unlike most other hazards, radiation exposure can adversely affect many future generations. The need for conservative management of all radiation sources is obvious. There are still many unknowns, and research on a wide front is urgently needed (1).

That rather lays it on the line. It is up to the scientists to guard and protect the public. Of course, most of them will attempt to do that for the protection of themselves and their families.

Now, when accidents do happen, how can panic be prevented? By avoiding any type of censorship and getting the facts to the people simply, and as quickly as possible. As you know, in an atomic mishap there seldom is danger except to those immediately involved at the installation. However, it is possible that there are hazards beyond the installation in that some atomic device or material may get where it does not belong. If there is a hazard, this should be stated. Say how great it is. Tell what precautions the public should take.

From the point of view of the press, this information should be telephoned to news media—newspapers, TV and radio—at once, and the steady flow of information about developments should continue until the story is completed from all angles. Be certain in advance that you have an administrative setup to handle information. One man should be available around the clock to give out concise, complete and factual information—again in simple language, so that everyone can understand.

Large plants and the government atomic complexes have trained publicity men who should do this automatically, but there are smaller organizations and research groups without such personnel. The small installations without public relations men must learn how and what media to contact. See to it that there are sufficient telephones available on which the media may recontact the mishap scene.

There are reassurances even in bad radiation accidents. The affected, with modern treatment, have good recovery chances. In news releases, the good as well as the bad should be brought out. The American public has never panicked when it knew the truth immediately. It is uncertainty that causes panic. You can give certainty or create uncertainty. The problem is yours, but the mass news media, given proper cooperation, stand ready to help.

REFERENCE

1. *The Biological Effects of Atomic Radiation.* National Academy of Sciences–National Research Council, Washington, D.C., 1960.

DISCUSSION

Mr. L. H. Cooper (Babcock & Wilcox Company, Ohio): I get a little shook up by the word "censored," and every reporter in the United States is not named Kleckner. I know I've heard a lot of publicity, and there is no question about it, he can keep things on an even keel, but I believe that, in the mass media, newspapers and television, controlled dissemination of facts is not necessarily censorship.

I gave a series of lectures to all volunteer fire departments in a very large area around Alliance, and I thought I had done it pretty well. The next night a TV program came on and it had to do with radiation, and without going into detail, everything was hot—the pump that put the gasoline in the automobile, and the horn button. It cancelled to a considerable extent everything that had been said. But I believe that if the press would stop using the word "censored" when they really don't mean that—because as far as I'm concerned, censoring is pulling the curtain down tight—if we could talk more about controlled dissemination, we could get away from some of the criticism that some of the smaller newspapers give these things in that they argue the public is supposed to know what the facts are. Now, the facts the public should know, in my opinion, are the ones that involve their safety and not the gory details some newspapers would prefer to print.

Mr. Kleckner: I think the gentleman got into a matter of terminology and semantics. I don't know whether you'd call it managed news or censorship. We don't want the gory details; we want the factual details, simply told. It may be true, and I know it is true, that some newspapers go all out for sensationalism. In Ohio, you have some good science writers who handle the facts straight. The major newspapers today, coast to coast, try to have men who are at least partially trained in the various fields.

Chairman Lanzl: I wonder if I could ask Mr. Unruh a question. Can radiation accidents go undetected for long periods?

Mr. Unruh: They certainly have, occasionally, but they should not. Careful emergency planning and proper engineering and design of the facilities should provide for early detection. The longer an accident or a near-accident condition goes undetected, the more chance there is that very serious events may occur. So I would hope that we would provide equipment to detect these things. Procedures and training should be provided so that people seeing an abnormal condition will be able to recognize it. Many times it is a case where something looks very common to an ordinary operator, whereas a physicist or health protection man in the area might quickly recognize that an abnormal condition exists.

This is part of the training program which we should get across to all people involved with radioactive materials.

Mr. Kleckner: Along that line, just two weeks ago I had a story from a doctor in suburban Washington. He is doing some particularly interesting work with contact lenses and has developed a double contact with an air space in it which can be worn for periods up to six hours. It was intended originally for scuba diving. They can be either blank or in the form of corrective lenses. They have had some success with the outer glass: when it is exposed to radiation, it will change colors. This conceivably can be developed into goggles to be worn by industrial and other atomic workers, to give them immediate notification that they themselves are being exposed.

Dr. R. K. Clark (Human Systems Institute, Chicago, Illinois): My comment concerns publicity of mishaps. As an emergency develops, one has multiple problems. One has to define the nature and extent of an emergency and institute appropriate procedures for its control. While he is working that out, the question arises, how soon should this information be made public? If he makes announcements too soon, he has to be conservative in order to prevent people from entering an area inappropriately. If he is making announcements hurriedly, he is apt to make it look bigger than it may be. Yet, if he waits and controls the information until he knows exactly what the facts are, this perhaps is a delay of twenty-four hours. Now, I don't know too much about news, but I have an impression that a twenty-four-hour delay can be taken as censorship.

Chapter II

INITIAL HANDLING OF EMERGENCIES AT THE SCENE

ACTIONS AT THE SITE OF A RADIATION ACCIDENT

MILO D. VOSS

Ames Laboratory, U.S. Atomic Energy Commission, and
Iowa State University
of Science and Technology
Ames, Iowa

OUR EXPERIENCE with radiation accidents runs the range from an SL-1 (Stationary Low Power Plant #1) reactor accident (1, 2, 3) to the loss of a few microcuries of carbon-14. Small accidental releases (spills) of radioactive materials are so commonplace as to give almost routine experience to health physicists in large atomic-energy installations. It is from such experience that one draws wisdom to extrapolate to actions for handling accidents in general.

For the purpose of this discussion, we shall consider actions which may be applicable, but which are not necessarily needed in all radiation emergency situations. This is necessary in order to present a generalized treatment of actions to be applied to particular situations. Upon careful consideration of accident potentials, it will be possible to relate these actions to your particular needs.

When specific action is called for to handle an emergency involving radiation or radioactive materials, the proper procedure is to activate the appropriate emergency organization. The ability to place in operation an organization, a team, or even one man requires that planning, staffing, and equipping have already been accomplished. The amount of assurance, poise, and effectiveness in handling emergency situations will depend upon the preparations which have been made in advance of the occurrence of an accident.

In making plans for coping with the various kinds of possible incidents, one must take into account the consequences of probable unwise acts and of operational and equipment failures. Based on this type of analysis, general actions may be planned which will provide reasonably effective countermeasures. Common-sense procedures will usually prove adequate. However, reactions of individuals at the time of an incident may not always be common-sense responses to the problem at hand. Instead, the inappropriate actions may increase exposures, hazards, and the effort required for control, restoration, and reclamation. Thorough preplanning, staffing and equipping, indoctrination, training, and practice will eliminate most of the bungling that comes with inexperience. It requires persistent effort to go from a paper plan to an effective operation. The training and practice necessary to assure some facility in coping with emergencies will be discussed.

It is my purpose to present a number of actions to be undertaken in response to or in defense against a variety of incidents which can occur in the use of radioactive materials and radiation. In each case, the general type of action as well as specific details are briefly discussed. Within this framework, actions applicable to most accidents are included; however, depending on the type and magnitude of an incident, not all of these will be necessary or desirable in a given situation.

The actions have been grouped according to: A) Incident Termination; B) Exposure Control; C) Medical Control; D) Support Actions, and E) Information. Actions for restoration and reclamation of facilities should not be considered by the same criteria as actions leading to control of the emergency.

A) ***Incident Termination*** actions involve the "victims" directly, and may also involve other persons.

Evacuation is the first step to be taken. Even though it may not be necessary in every case, if an alarm sounds calling for that action—*Go!* Prompt response may be life-saving. The magnitude of evacuation necessary depends upon the nature of the occurrence and on the hazard level. Leaving a room may suffice in one case and in another, abandoning a building and going to a considerable distance from it may be necessary.

Along with evacuation, *assembly and retention* of personnel must be considered. To be released to go home or to wander about may bring hazards to others or cause further damage to the victim. Immediate release may also make other efforts, such as exposure control and medical control, more difficult.

Where and when it is required, some shut-down of the affected facility may be advisable. The spread of contamination may be prevented by turning off or reducing ventilation. Turning off heaters, electrical machines, and running water may help contain the accident and prevent additional mishaps. In the case of radiation generators, it may be possible to terminate an incident by turning off the power supply. Although it is not always the case, machines which utilize a high potential, as well as neutron generators, under some conditions, may have residual radiations.

Suppression and containment may be useful. Covering a spill with absorbent material, spreading a heavy foam agent, or simply shutting a door may prevent the spread of radioactivity. The dispersal of settled contamination into the air must always be guarded against.

Rescue operations may need to be undertaken. A victim of radioactive contamination and radiation exposure may also have received injuries which make him unable to move or care for himself. Prompt decisions and speedy actions are essential if rescue is to be effective. A weighty problem in connection with rescue operations must be faced. If the limits for the emergency exposure of rescue personnel have been reached, abandonment of the injured must be accepted as a principle of operation.

A *personnel accounting* must be made as promptly as possible. Preparation for this problem beforehand may prevent much confusion and distress, should a serious accident occur. In order to provide appropriate care and reassurance to families, it is necessary to know where all involved individuals were at the time of the accident. This may not be easy in some cases. In installations where serious accidents are possible, continuous personnel accounting may need to be considered. All persons involved in emergency operations must also be accounted for at all times. Suitable identification for these people will be helpful where their recognition is important. In order to establish effective exposure control for emergency personnel, the latter must have their accumulated dose recorded. The accounting for evacuated personnel and the rescue of exposed and injured personnel complete the direct actions to be taken to terminate the incident. However, many aspects of an accident can still be considered to be of an emergency nature, even after the termination of rescue activities.

B) ***Exposure Control*** is another action to be taken. The exposure of individuals who were direct victims of external irridiation or who are engaged in emergency operations should be reduced or terminated. Personnel may be subject to various degrees of radioactive contamination. *Decontamination* of personnel is, therefore, an urgent order of business to reduce or terminate exposure. Decontamination may involve removal of contaminated clothing, spot washing, or more drastic efforts. Contaminated wounds and internal contamination present special problems of an emergency nature which are not likely to be handled at the scene. Besides maintaining control of exposure to external radiation, *respiratory protection* and protection against further contamination of emergency personnel must be provided.

In the event that a contaminating incident has occurred, or a radiation field has been created, the contamination *site must be defined* by surveying and sampling operations. If the site of the accident and of its effects is confined to areas under the control of plant or facility management, many problems are eliminated. If, on the other hand, contamination has spread to adjacent areas including private and community property, the problems may be serious indeed. Evacuation of these areas and the denial of their use may be needed to control exposure of neighbors.

Access limitation may be necessary. It may be sufficient to close the accident area by labeling a doorway or, in more serious cases, to establish check points about the area. The areas of limited access must be changed as reclamation proceeds. Restrictions should remain in effect until the radiation has been reduced to non-emergency levels, or until decontamination has been accomplished.

Monitoring and survey operations are necessary to determine the extent of personnel radiation exposure and area contamination. Surveys will provide the basis for determining the cleanup operations to be undertaken. Personnel monitoring and dose rate assessment will provide information for possible medical treatment. Measurements of air concentrations will help to define the areas affected by radioactive releases to the environment.

Administrative control must be established early in the operation. Control functions, access limitation, surveying and coordination of effort cannot be accomplished without someone in authority. In some instances, administrative control is readily achieved. It may be difficult in cases where an accident has occurred on private property, or on public property containing material of different ownership the responsibility for which may not be clear. As an example of such an area of uncertainty, let us consider that a shipment of cobalt-60 from a supplier to a purchaser over public roads by a common carrier is involved in an accident; fire breaks out, resulting in contamination. This radiation problem demands an administrative decision. Who is responsible at this point? Effective administrative and operational control is needed to prevent additional radiation exposures.

C) ***Medical Control*** and assistance for persons who have received substantial radiation exposures is necessary. First aid operations may be required at the accident site. Preliminary screening also may be accomplished at or near the site. The amount of contamination of wounds or abrasions must be measured. Where large numbers of people are involved, dosimetric screening will help to show who needs attention, and in what order. Little more than this can be done at the site.

D) ***Support Actions*** may include a substantial effort in some cases, while relatively little may be needed in others. A contaminated person with injuries may require the services of an ambulance for transportation; evacuation of a plant may require considerably more in the way of transportation and drivers.

Outside assistance may be needed. The Atomic Energy Commission Emergency Assistance Teams are a source of help. Specialists or persons experienced in radiation emergencies should be on call for aid. State police, firemen, and local Civil Defense organizations may be willing and able to offer assistance.

E) ***Information*** is included as an action. It is best to avoid using the word "control" in this instance, even though control over the dissemination of information may be needed. Information in this sense includes communications and the development of data.

There will be *reporting requirements* that must be met. The management of the facility where the accident occurred, the state, and the Atomic Energy Commission will need accident reports.

Information releases to the news media will need to be made. A single responsible person should have the authority to release information. Conflicting, inaccurate, incomplete or unqualified statements may do a great deal of damage, both during an emergency period and in the later operational periods, and even after recovery is complete.

Internal communication and control are necessary. The fullest and most accurate communication must be maintained during operations of an emergency nature. To have less than full knowledge by all people involved is to invite trouble. Sessions may be needed to provide general and detailed information on proposed operations; this will avoid misunderstandings while such operations are being carried out.

Data and records must be kept on all aspects of the emergency operations. Information will be needed for an evaluation of operations, and for later review. Records may be needed for various legal requirements at a later date.

Some twenty specific actions associated with the scene or site of an emergency have been given. The planning and action used in a given instance should be suitable for the operation involved. Accidents may occur with radiation machines, sealed sources, unsealed radioisotopes, and nuclear reactors; in industries, universities, hospitals, and government laboratories; with on-site or off-site effects. To have suitable actions planned and ready when they are needed should be the goal, and proper preparation will provide the capability to handle any emergency which may arise.

REFERENCES

1. Pittman, Frank: AEC's Pittman Reports on the SL-1 Accident. *Nucleonics, 19*:No. 3, 62-9, 1961.
2. *SL-1 Accident.* Atomic Energy Commission Investigation Board Report, Joint Committee on Atomic Energy of the U.S. Congress, U.S. Government Printing Office, Washington, D.C., p. 173, June 1961.
3. SL-1 Explosion Kills 3; Cause and Significance Still Unclear. *Nucleonics, 19*:No. 2, 17-23, 1961.

MENTAL PREPAREDNESS OF EMERGENCY PERSONNEL

DONALD OKEN

Michael Reese Hospital
Chicago, Illinois

RADIATION ACCIDENTS are an unfamiliar area for a psychiatrist. Yet, I need not feel entirely out of place. Psychiatrists and radiation scientists do share in common a somewhat similar public image. Both of us may be seen as Rasputin-like characters who, clad in black robes inscribed with crescents and stars, inhabit dark places where we deal with the vile mysteries of occult forces.

In one way, I must fall in with a related type of image, namely that of the psychiatrist as a fortune teller. For my discussion is based on no direct experience whatsoever with radiation incidents. Nor, unfortunately, is there much information available about the psychological aspects of such incidents. There is, however, a fairly large body of knowledge from related areas which can be meaningfully extrapolated to the problem under consideration. Moreover, I believe that this material can be applied in a practical way. I do not intend to remain at the level of high-flown theory, though I shall base my discussion on theory as well as experimental data.

Let me add a few words to demarcate my approach further. My experience, as a psychiatrist, has to do with the treatment of individuals and small groups. Here, however, it is more appropriate to concentrate on issues which should be subsumed under the words "management" or "effective handling" rather than "treatment." Our concern also is with issues relevant to larger, less well-defined groups. These include not only members of a particular emergency team, but also emergency personnel generally, and even the public at large. What I shall say has relevance to incidents of various magnitudes. But I shall make no attempt to deal with issues specifically related to the mass-scale disasters of nuclear war which are not the concern here (although I shall draw on some of the observations made at Hiroshima and Nagasaki (9)).

Anxiety

Radiation accidents involve the threat of great danger. Our initial attention is directed, therefore, to the phenomenon of anxiety which constitutes the normal biological response to psychologically stressful conditions.

The concept of anxiety is central in psychiatric theory. Anxiety is viewed as a signal which heralds threat and sets in motion a variety of psychosomatic processes designed to maintain the integrity of the organism. On the psychological side, there is a searching out and processing of sensory stimuli which are reviewed against the background of memory traces and subjected to cognitive analysis. This provides an estimate of the source, nature, and extent of the threat. It also results in the institution of both "defenses" which maintain psychological integration, and overt behavioral responses which are directed to effect mastery of the environment. Concomitantly, a variety of physiological processes is set in motion. These include changes which produce the familiar physical symptoms of anxiety: increased heart rate, blood pressure, and respiratory exchange; pupillary dilation; sweating; etc. There are also silent internal changes which include an elevation of blood sugar, enhanced blood coagulability, shunting of the circulation from the viscera to the muscles, and others. In a series of now classic researches carried out during the 1920's, W. B. Cannon (1) demonstrated that these changes are largely the result of a generalized discharge of the sympathetic nervous system and adrenalin release. Further, he pointed out their great adaptive value in preparing an organism for "fight or flight." At moderate levels of anxiety, the organism is vigilant and is alertly searching its environment, prepared to deal rapidly and effectively with its internal stress responses or with needs for appropriate behavioral response, i.e., it is superbly mobilized.

From an evolutionary standpoint (as Hamburg (6) has discussed), preparation for physical action was entirely appropriate in the primitive world of tooth and claw. For modern man, life is very different. Many stresses require subtle and delicate adaptational adjustments, which may be entirely psychological in nature with no need for action. Everyone is familiar with the restlessness which occurs at times of increased tensions. Anxiety produces a marked impulsion to act. Conversely, action tends to relieve anxiety. Naturally, the most effective action is that which successfully resolves the stress situation. But, just as inactivity itself may be stressful, almost any kind of activity makes one feel better. Simply doing something—anything—provides a sense of mastery which (combined with its distracting effects) provides great relief from anxiety.

Thus far, we have considered milder forms of anxiety. At high levels, anxiety is no longer adaptive. More intense threats overwhelm the readily available mechanisms of defense. More primitive, pathological defenses are called emergently into play, and these distort the perception of reality. Higher personality functions are sacrificed. Perceptual discriminations break down in the panicky scanning of the environment, resulting in an inability to separate benign or helpful cues from threats. Everything in the environment becomes a danger. Gaps in information, augmented by the existing intellectual confusion, become filled with fearsome fantasies. A last-ditch defensive blocking out of all stimuli may occur, resulting in a stunned, trance-like state ot psychological paralysis. A sense of helplessness supervenes, akin to the feeling of a small child. Many of these changes become self-reinforcing in a circular fashion, leading to a mounting crescendo of terror. Moreover, as defenses and intellectual functions fail, the ensuing sense of personality disintegration and unreality becomes the source of further anxiety.

This extreme picture is very uncommon. Rarely, one encounters it in an unusually severe psychiatric illness or in situations of extreme stress such as the battlefield (4). Nevertheless, it is essential to know the full-blown picture thoroughly. A few individuals may develop terror or become abjectly dazed if they are closely affected by a major radiation incident. Almost everyone involved will develop some anxiety. And whenever anxiety occurs, most of the phenomena described will occur, albeit in an attenuated and partial form.

In such a situation, all emergency personnel should be prepared to apply energetic therapeutic measures. I have already indicated the similarity of the anxious adult to the helpless, bewildered state of a frightened small child. As with the child, the only voice which can be heard is that of a parent-like figure, whose strength communicates an omnipotent ability to control danger and whose warm concern (love) insures that such action will be taken. Personnel should take pains to be warm, supportive, and interested. Team members should be able to work in a calm, competent manner which communicates confidence, not anxiety. Help should be provided as if the team knew exactly what it was doing—as, indeed, it should. Material aid is, itself, very reassuring; but active verbal reassurance is essential, too. All communications are best kept simple and to the point. Repetition is also of great importance. Only in this way can one break through the confusion. Reassurances are best made as specific as possible, and related to the immediate needs of the victim, for anxiety is right now. Information should be provided to fill in gaps of knowledge and to serve as a corrective for fantasied fears. Again, it should be concrete, simple, repetitive, and related specifically to the immediate situation. When an individual learns that he is well taken care of by able, interested people who can clarify his ideas about the real dangers and how they can be dealt with, his anxiety will drop. At this point he can begin to reconstitute his own defenses more effectively. This is a good time to enlist his aid in carrying out simple activities to assist himself and others.

Overall, this approach can be expected to be effective in dealing with the great majority of stress reactions encountered at the scene. It will also have a useful preventative role, for, without help, even milder stress responses may develop into chronic anxiety states or other forms of persistent psychiatric disorder.

The Strange and Unknown

Situations which are psychologically stressful fall into three general categories. These are the threats of: 1) physical harm; 2) loss of love and security, and 3) separation from loved ones. It is clear that all of these may be the consequences of a radiation incident. Each person will be more or less vulnerable to a specific situation depending on the way in which he interprets the situation in terms of these threat categories and upon his general psychological (ego) strength.

There are two additional major factors which define the existence and intensity of stress. One can be described by the words unexpectedness, novelty, or strangeness. The other relates to vagueness and ambiguity. Man's need for a world characterized by predictability, dependability, and clarity is very strong.

The importance of these factors was well demonstrated in one of our early stress experiments (11). An initial, pre-experimental "control" session in our psychosomatic laboratory led to major psychological and physiological stress effects which exceeded the response on subsequent experimental stress days. This occurred because of the exposure to an unfamiliar laboratory full of strange equipment, in which there was no way to know what to expect, even though "nothing really happened." Additional confirmation comes from a study of the effects of bombings during World War II, by Janis (9). "Variable and wide intervals between successive raids tend to have a more disturbing effect than regular short intervals."

In general, repetition of stress situations has a progressively attenuated effect, as familiarization occurs. Contributing to this is the learning of techniques of defense which become more readily available with practice. There is, however, one crucial proviso. The "practice" must be reasonably successful. When stress is so severe that massive anxiety is aroused (what we refer to as an acutely traumatic situation), the learning which occurs is that the situation must be avoided at all cost. Subsequent exposure to that stress, or even milder reminders, may produce full-blown terror. This is well illustrated by the responses of soldiers with combat reactions who, for days after being removed from combat, leap for cover at any loud noise (4). The prevention of this type of traumatic reaction by familiarization is highly relevant. We shall have cause to refer to it later.

Let us return to a consideration of strangeness and ambiguity. Both have an important bearing on the radiation problem. Even to the scientifically sophisticated, radiation is a complex phenomenon with many hidden qualities, and one with great power. For the layman, these strange, unclear qualities are magnified a thousandfold. Radiation is an invisible, silent, intangible, seemingly unpredictable force of mysterious nature, which has the magical capacity to produce effects at a distance without apparent cause. Its potential power and destructiveness are beyond real comprehension. Little wonder that it is regarded with awe and dread! And little wonder that the radiation scientist is cast in the role which I half-jokingly described earlier.

One of our prime tasks, therefore, is to provide a more concrete, tangible, realistic, familiar "image" of radiation and of its effects. I shall offer two possible approaches. We might emphasize the particulate nature of radiation, dealing with it as a concrete and tangible thing. Its invisibility then can be explained in terms of its small size. (Dimension itself is familiar and implies the realness of that which is measured.) One problem with this approach is a possible tendency to interpret radiation effects as being like bullets striking a target. However, this destructive implication can be surmounted as, for example, in the explanation of chemotherapeutic drugs as "magic bullets."

A second approach might be to consider radiation as being like a more powerful form of sunlight. While sunlight is not really a tangible phenomenon (and it is far from simple or fully understood), it is very familiar and benign. With this approach, biological radiation effects can be seen as something like sunburn (which is not too far off): a phenomenon which is familiar, is tangible, and is viewed as basically good, though dangerous when overdone. The heat and power of reactors, and even explosion effects, might be explained as being like the effects of a magnifying glass.

I do not wish to belabor either suggestion. Both are presented as examples only. The point is that we must develop a model of radiation which can be made into a reified, tangible, comprehensible thing, with primarily good qualities, which is reasonably consistent with our scientific concepts. We must communicate this effectively and often enough to the public and to personnel, so that the idea not only gets through, but that radiation becomes a familiar everyday matter, thus losing its mystery.

Let me emphasize that this type of model of radiation should find usefulness in the work of emergency personnel dealing with an incident. At such a time, it is absolutely essential that personnel talk and act in a manner consistent with this kind of model. That fact must be made a part of their training. At a more primary level, they *themselves* must hold such an attitude. There is no point in trying to communicate something which you yourself don't believe: doubt is transmitted very clearly. It should be remembered, too, that emergency personnel start out by being members of the "public." If we wish them to function effectively, they cannot be hampered by their own frightened fantasies about radiation.

Group Psychology

The focus, thus far, has been on the individual. Let us turn to a consideration of the psychology of groups (3). The ties which hold a group together center about their mutual allegiance to shared purposes, goals and ideals, and to their common leadership. Stated in psychiatric terms, the group members have developed an *identification* with one another. As individuals work closely together over time, the body of their shared experiences mounts steadily to strengthen their identification. Group traditions cement this, as do developing bonds of respect and affection. When we talk about *morale,* what we refer to is the strength of these ties among group members: to one another and to their leaders. Through these ties, each individual "borrows" the strength of the group as a shield against anxiety. Members of a group with high morale thus become capable of carrying out tasks which are personally unappealing or even severely stressful.

The group also sets a norm as to how much anxiety is acceptable and how it may be expressed. Soldiers in combat, for example, may admit to a certain degree of internal fear. They can gripe about the food and discomfort, the enemy, and the support troops. But disparagement of the unit itself or self-protective avoidance of responsibilities to one's buddies is intolerable. So is uncontrollable anxiety. Individuals who transgress these limits must be excluded. If many are retained, they become a source of disintegration for the group as a whole. Morale plummets. This kind of phenomenon is one central feature in group panic, as in the case when a whole combat unit flees its sector. It is not just that anxiety (as any emotion) tends to spread contagiously by means of the empathy which characterizes human beings. What occurs, also, is that the sight of one individual in flight is a signal that the group ties have failed for him, indicating to the next man that these are not so strong and protective. He, then, becomes more vulnerable and flees also; and the process spreads. However, the likelihood of group panic is much overrated. Panic is rare, even in extreme stress (2). Little was seen at Hiroshima or

Nagasaki (9). Other determinants besides stress are responsible for its occurrence.

The leader is, far and away, the most important person in the group. If he should reveal feet of clay, the effects are disastrous. Remember how, in our recent national crisis, we turned to President Johnson. His ability to demonstrate strength and continuity of leadership was vital. All of us, I believe, had a distinct feeling for several days that the very national survival hinged on his slightest move.

Obviously, team leaders must be chosen with great care. It is difficult, however, to specify how this is to be done. Just what is leadership? It is far more than knowing concretely what to do. It rests centrally on the capacity to attract allegiance from others, giving them the feeling that the leader will always take proper care of them. The best predictor is the past. Men who have demonstrated proven leadership ability are the best bet. But it is very difficult to predict with real consistency who will demonstrate leadership qualities when a new situation demands them.

During a radiation disaster, all emergency personnel become leaders. Partly, this is a function of their work. But they are, as well, the embodiment and representative of larger authority. Hence, it becomes essential that they understand this role. Training for the entire emergency team must make them aware of this, as well as of the underlying basis in group psychology.

Selection and Training

Of course, other abilities are necessary, also. The most important is the capacity to withstand the stresses which will be faced in the course of carrying out effective function. Those who have successfully mastered other stresses will, generally, stand up best. The wider the range of these stresses and the more these overlap with stresses which will occur, the more dependable is this criterion. Experience dictates, however, that selection has a very limited value. Moreover, the common assumption that this means the winnowing out of the neurotic is false. Many "neurotics" have served with distinction in our country's wars. And who among us is not somewhat neurotic? Everyone has different points of strength and vulnerability.

If selection offers little help, training provides ample means to take up this slack. This can be stated with assurance. Fortunately, we know a good deal about the factors involved. First are those lessons which come from our knowledge of group psychology. Emergency teams must be suffused with a strong *esprit de corps*. Every effort should be made to inculcate a sense of group unity. Shared activities should be pushed, even in areas of recreation. But group demarcation is not enough. Members should be imbued with the feeling that the group is something special: that they are an elite, the chosen. The Atomic Energy Commission personnel have a headstart here. The agency already has achieved select status. Industrial teams will have a harder job. A uniform, insignia or badge may help. Special procedures, such as the trappings of secrecy, need not be ignored as being too childish. Incentives and rewards should be provided. Do not mistake this as implying material privilege. Think, for example, of the remarkable morale of the Marines. This is based primarily on their notion of being tougher than others, and being more willing to endure hardship.

Training should be carried out as a unit, preferably directed by the same men who will continue to serve as leaders. While small unit cohesiveness is emphasized, allegiance to the larger group must be maintained. Ideals and long-term goals should be stressed constantly. These provide a bridge of strength when the individual is isolated. Planning decisions will dictate specific variations. For example, emphasis on geographical loyalties must be balanced against plans for a mobile team to be used far from its home base. Possibly, unit formation should be based on functional lines. Thus, if fire-fighters were called to one area and the medical team to another, neither would experience group fragmentation. Other variations will suggest themselves as needed.

Our knowledge of anxiety also provides important help in planning training procedures. You recall that stress mastery is enhanced by past successful experience. Thus, our first job is to anticipate what stresses will occur. We should then include exposure to these stresses in training. But this is to be planned as a graded exposure, with slow increments of stress intensity and demand for performance. Early team training should include, for example, the bandaging of one another. Training films should precede direct exposure to injured human beings. Severe wounds or burns should be viewed only after minor injuries have been seen. This approach develops stress tolerance as well as technical competence, and prevents the occurrence of an acutely traumatic response.

Later stages of training should include practical work at real disasters. Floods, fires, train wrecks and the like will provide valuable experience with many similarities to the radiation incidents later to be faced. Simulated practical exercises also can help. The capacity for the men to mobilize themselves for action and the effectiveness with which they work then can be observed. Every simulated or real incident should be subjected to a thorough "Monday morning quarter-backing" by the entire unit. Films of actual performance can be very helpful. Carried out in the spirit of helping the group to achieve top skills, rather than as adverse criticism, these sessions will serve to weld the team together and enhance its sense of superiority. Follow-up reviews and the training drills themselves have the added advantage of filling in gaps of time. Nothing is so destructive to morale as periods of prolonged inactivity. This is another reason for using teams in non-radiation situations or in minor radiation incidents which could be handled by operational personnel alone.

Some Further Issues

I would like to turn now, very briefly, to some additional areas which are relevant to my general topic. The first is the role of *information.* Earlier I mentioned the tendency for an anxious individual to fill in perceptual gaps with fearful fantasies. The analogous process which develops in the group situation is rumor (5). (Nature abhors a vacuum in the psychological as much as in the physical world.) The number of rumors and their frightfulness will be a function of the absence of realistic information and of the extent of anxiety. Scare stories rapidly circulate through an anxious group, acting to stimulate still more anxiety. The antidote is information. Even if the news is bad, it is always reassuring to realize that you know the worst. Emergency teams, therefore, should be supplied with a maximum of correct information and trained in the most helpful methods of communicating this to victims. The crucial role of information also suggests the value of having information specialists as part of a disaster team. Victims of an incident may be said to include those in the surrounding community, often within a wide radius, who have heard that an "atomic disaster" has occurred.

Second, let us turn to the question of *prevention*. This is the logical place where one really should begin to deal with accidents. There are ample data indicating that most "accidents" are motivated acts subserving psychological needs. I do not, however, base my concern on data derived from other situations only. A review of reports of past criticality and reactor incidents (7) and discussions held with some of the health personnel in charge reveal a number of striking peculiarities in the behavior of many of those involved—in which they almost literally asked for trouble. This has occurred in the face of an Atomic Energy Commission safety program which has been pushed hard and has generally been highly effective. We know that some individuals have a particular psychological make-up leading to frequent accidents. These "accident-prone" (10) people sometimes can be identified on psychological grounds. A far better predictor is their history of previous accidents. It seems evident, then, that the selection of scientists and personnel for sensitive work should include screening for this factor.

More recently, it has become apparent that accidents tend to occur in clusters during periods in which other signs of psychological stress are evident—the "accident process" or "accident syndrome" (8). Usually, many behavioral signs precede the major accident. There are two inferences to be drawn from this. Workers who show signs of psychological tension or sudden changes in behavior, especially if they have a series of minor accidents, should be scrutinized by health personnel. And certainly it is advisable for anyone who has had one serious accident to be examined carefully before he returns to work. Some form of psychiatric treatment might be indicated. Perhaps every installation should have, as a part of its health division, a psychiatrist or psychologist.

We should remember, too, that even scientists are not immune to anxious fantasies about the nature of radiation. Nor are they immune to handling these by a technique of defense which we call *denial*, i.e., acting as if danger did not exist. Denial is especially prone to occur when a threat is vague and intense. Both qualities can be attributed to radiation all too readily. Denial is a highly effective defense, but a dangerously maladaptive one which may lead to carelessness or an unrealistic taking of chances. A sustained safety educational program must continually be emphasized for all personnel.

Finally, I would like to point out that we still have much to learn. If I have seemed often to deal with generalities in this paper, this is not entirely because of its broad subject matter. When there are few specific data, one is restricted to the application of broad principles. And there are very few data. The topics which I have discussed, and many others which are related, provide fertile and important areas for research. If we are to progress further, it is essential that this be pursued energetically.

REFERENCES

1. Cannon, W. B.: *Bodily Changes in Pain, Hunger, Fear and Rage.* D. Appleton & Company, New York, 1927.
2. Fritz, C. E., and Marks, E. S.: The NORC Studies of Human Behavior in Disaster. *J. Social Issues, 10*:No. 3, 1954.
3. Freud, S.: *Group Psychology and the Analysis of the Ego,* Tr. by T. Strachey. Liveright, New York, 1940.
4. Grinker, R. R., and Spiegel, J. P.: *Men Under Stress.* Blakiston, Philadelphia, 1945.
5. Grinker, R. R.: Anxiety as a Significant Variable for a Unified Theory of Human Behavior. *Arch. Gen. Psychiat., 1*:537-46, 1959.
6. Hamburg, D.: Relevance of Recent Evolutionary Changes to Human Stress Biology, unpublished manuscript. Delivered at the Conference on Social Life of Early Man, Burg Wartenstein, Austria, June 1959.
7. Hayes, D. F.: A Summary of Accidents and Incidents Involving Radiation in Atomic Energy Activities, June 1945 through December 1955. U.S. Atomic Energy Commission, Oak Ridge, 1956 (plus Supplements: August 1957, September 1959, and December 1961).
8. Hirschfeld, A. H., and Behan, R. C.: The Accident Process; I. Etiological Considerations of Industrial Injuries. *J.A.M.A., 186*:193-199, 1963.
9. Janis, I. L.: *Air War and Emotional Stress.* McGraw-Hill Book Company, New York, 1951.
10. Rawson, A. J.: Accident Proneness. *Psychosom. Med., 6*:86-94, 1944.
11. Sabshin, M., Hamburg, D. A., Grinker, R. R., Persky, H., Basowitz, H., Korchin, S., and Chevalier, J.: Significance of Pre-experimental Studies in the Psychosomatic Laboratory. *A.M.A. Arch. Neurol. Psychiat., 78*: 207, 1957.

SCREENING RADIOACTIVELY EXPOSED PERSONS FOR MEDICAL ATTENTION, DECONTAMINATION OR RELEASE

JOHN H. PINGEL

*Argonne National Laboratory**
Argonne, Illinois

IN ANY EMERGENCY there is an order in which things are done. In a general way, this order can be preset. The emergency worker is guided in establishing the sequence of actions to be taken by concepts and ideas which rule his thinking and actions in an emergency situation. The quality of his performance and the completeness of fulfillment of the objectives of emergency action depend on a number of factors:

1) The quality and excellence of the concepts, beliefs, and ideas by which he operates.

2) The completeness with which such concepts and ideas rule the emergency worker. This, in turn, depends on such things as the degree of training of the individual; the thoroughness with which he knows and believes in the rightness of the ideas and of the action pattern; the experience which he has in using the concepts and ideas—the practice of the action pattern; the capability of the individual to handle and use the materials and things involved, including the radiation safety equipment; the general store of experience and technical knowledge of the individual; and the alertness and sensitiveness of the individual to the needs of the moment.

3) The quality and quantity (adequacy) of radiation safety materials (instruments, clothes changes, protective equipment, etc.) on hand, and the capability of the emergency workers to use such materials to best advantage.

4) The degree to which the accident situation needs are fulfilled by trained persons who can fully assume responsibility to act to the

*Operated by the University of Chicago for the U.S. Atomic Energy Commission.

best of their ability to render aid, and who can freely act in the name of the organ (plant, company, government unit) involved.

In most accident or emergency situations, the following general order of action ideas is prescribed and followed:

1) People must be cared for first.

2) Next, the accident scene should be gotten under control. This includes stopping fires, preventing further exposures, delineating, containing, and preventing spread of contamination (movement of people and movement of air are the two chief sources of the spread of contamination), and saving equipment and materials from destruction, if possible, without endangering lives.

3) Restorative measures should be carried on in a calm and careful manner.

Screening is only a passing phase of accident handling, but requires specialized knowledge and training in persons who handle accident situations. Screening of victims (persons wounded, irradiated, or contaminated, including clothing contamination) takes place as the first order of business in handling accidents and emergencies, as it is the phase of taking care of people. It is a phase of evacuation, prevention of further exposure, prevention of spread of contamination, and handling of accident victims.

Ideally, the screening of victims should accomplish the following: a) that released persons will not have received serious exposure and will know what to do about insignificant levels of radioactive contamination that they may be allowed to carry off on their bodies and clothing; b) that seriously injured or radioactively exposed individuals are given promptly into the hands of capable medical personnel; c) that persons with lesser injuries and radiation exposures are also turned over to the care of medical personnel with the knowledge of the extent of exposure; d) that all information regarding personnel exposures and accident assessment is given to medical personnel as soon as possible; e) that persons with contaminated clothing or bodies are informed as to what to do and expect, and are turned over to a decontamination team to be given clothes changes and to be decontaminated as soon as possible, and f) that all possible radiation exposures are measured with reasonable accuracy.

Screening takes place in several stages and in several locations. It includes gross rapid screening done immediately after an accident and very close to the accident scene, medical screening (triage, if necessary), screening at the decontamination station (the sorting out of difficult from easy cases), screening of emergency and decontamination workers who move into and out of the accident area, and screening of materials and equipment which are moved from the accident scene.

I. Gross Rapid Screening

For each accident handler who appears on the scene, there is an initial step during which he learns what has happened—in enough detail so that he can act intelligently with respect to the objectives. Then there is a short period of mental adjustment during which a decision to act, and possibly a brief plan of the type of action, is made. For late arrivers, the action decided on may simply be to volunteer to help. The expert emergency team worker has in mind training ideas and experience which, together with what he finds out about the accident, help him to work with effectiveness. The knowledge which the screener should have is discussed later.

Gross rapid screening has to be done without much delay, often without sufficient information. Hence it is almost always followed up by refining and completing processes such as more accurate dosimetry, more detailed examination of related information, bioassay sampling, recording and filling in those details which are unimportant in the initial press of getting the job done.

Gross screening is *defined* here as the orderly, knowledgeable process of rapidly evaluating the degree of injury and contamination involvement of persons coming from an accident scene, and the classifying and sending of such persons into treatment channels. It includes sending the victims to treatment stations with a clear understanding (if reasonably possible) as to what restorative measures, if any, are to take place.

The *objectives of emergency action* should normally be set according to the basic purpose leading to the formation of an emergency team or organ. They usually include the saving of lives, prevention of further exposure, containment, abatement, delineation and controlling of the accident to whatever degree and kind is applicable. These objectives should be very clearly thought out, written down, and learned by each member of the emergency organ. Thus, there can be a oneness of purpose and objective, and a resulting teamwork that is intelligent, effective, direct, purposeful and economical in time, effort and material.

The *general aim of gross screening* is:

1) To separate the victims into classes:
   a) Wounded.
   b) Wounded and contaminated.
   c) Those radioactively exposed to whom medical treatment or close observation is due.
   d) Those radioactively exposed who should be kept under observation, but for whom treatment may not be necessary (the victims may be hospitalized for observation, or held momentarily for clinical observation including bioassay sampling).
   e) Those contaminated externally—clothing, hair, body.
   f) Those non-exposed, non-contaminated.

2) To provide information concerning radiation and radioactivity exposure, contamination levels, and the nature of the exposure, to medical and decontamination personnel so that they can carry out their functions rapidly and effectively.

3) To send victims promptly to treatment stations with information on findings, including name, accident description, survey results, exposure information such as type of exposure, radionuclides involved, external contamination levels, likelihood of internal exposure, air sampling results, etc.

The *location* of the gross screening activity is normally the control point. The site should have or be made to have: a) one or more telephones; b) control of access to the site of the accident, so that all personnel going in can be checked for usefulness, proper equipment and clothing, and so that all persons leaving can be checked for injuries and contamination, and can be asked for bioassay samples; and c) access to emergency supplies. (See Figure II-1.)

In no radiation accidents except very minor ones is screening ever done at the scene. This is to prevent further exposure which is almost always likely to some degree at the accident scene. Screening is done

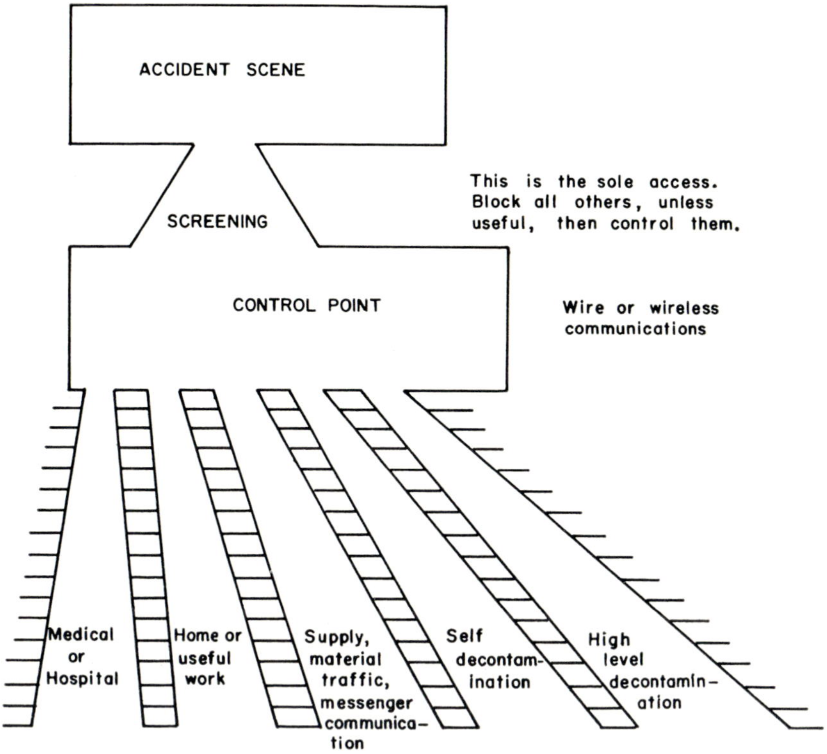

FIGURE II-1. Schematic Drawing of Effective Handling for Radiation Accidents.

as close to the scene as is reasonably possible. This is done to prevent spreading the contamination any further than necessary, and to have immediate contact with the accident scene in all phases of handling.

All traffic to and from the accident scene is controlled, and people and materials going in and out are surveyed for contamination. The gross rapid screening is generally done by health physicists and health physics technicians. As in the case of any other kind of accident, if a physician is needed he is called by persons at the scene. The health physicist's training should be such as to enable him to make this decision. It is wise for a clear understanding to exist between health physics personnel and medical personnel as to what kind of patients the physician wants to see. This will be discussed further under action levels (see p. 56 and p. 280).

For most small accidents, gross screening is an integral part of the initial accident handling procedure. Only when several surveyors are present and more than a few persons are exposed, or if contamination is widespread, is a special screening point designated. It is essential that screening be done immediately, with assurance and intelligence. This is difficult to do once people have scattered.

The *job of gross screening* involves one or more aspects:

1) A fast evaluation of an accident situation is often necessary so that screening personnel know what to look for. Information can be gotten from the persons involved in the accident, from preliminary measurements of radiation levels, from air and contamination surveys, and from pre-accident knowledge about the operation. The type of exposure must be determined before screening can be done readily. The types of exposure may be about as follows:

- a) Exposure to radiation only, such as x-rays, gamma radiation, beta radiation, accelerator radiations, neutrons, and criticality radiations consisting of mixtures of neutrons and gamma rays.
- b) Contamination exposures which usually include radiation exposure, but often in very small amounts.
- c) Exposure to combinations of the above.

Exposures can be to radioactive substances such as gases and aerosols, liquids, solids, dusts, explosions, surface contaminants and so on, as well as to radiation.

2) Screening includes first taking care of personnel with serious non-radiation injuries. It is a rule to do this *first,* regardless of what the radiation or contamination exposure is. One of the ways in which a radiation accident differs from ordinary accidents is that it is sometimes necessary to move the victims away from the scene of occurrence, even if they are seriously injured. However, before this is done, some decision needs to be made as to whether the effect of moving might not be more serious than further radiation exposure. This decision must be made immediately on the basis of measurements made at the scene. A physician should make the decision, if possible.

3) Screening involves collection of information or samples for dosage estimates. Careful records should be kept as to names of persons, locations of persons and materials collected, all instrument readings, instruments used, and pertinent time and duration of readings. This includes the following procedures:

a) Collecting all dosimeters and reading them immediately, if possible, collecting all information connecting the dosimeter and its location with the individuals and their locations at the time of the accident. If indium foils or other foils (provided for determining the neutron dose rapidly and roughly) are present, the required readings of these are taken. Then the dosimeters must be sent on their way to be evaluated.

b) Taking radiation readings at the places where persons received exposure, if this can be done safely; interviewing the persons involved (see questionnaire Appendix II-4) to establish the duration of the exposure. Often, dosage estimates can be made on the spot from such information. Dosage estimates are needed to screen out victims having received significant radiation exposures.

c) Making and recording contamination surveys of clothing and exposed body parts. Measurements at the nostrils and mouth often make it possible to get a rough idea as to whether or not internal exposure took place. Having the individual blow his nose can give a rough idea as to exposure to air contamination if the tissue is measured. However, these measurements do not necessarily constitute positive evidence that internal exposure has been received. The individual may have wiped his nose or face with contaminated hands.

d) If possible, determining the radionuclides involved. One must be cautious about relying completely on pre-accident knowledge, unless control of such information is exceptionally good. If the radionuclides are unknown, it is wise to collect a few samples which might later be analyzed.

e) Arranging for collection of bioassay samples. What samples are to be collected will have to be determined from knowledge obtained at the scene or available beforehand. If the type and severity of exposure (inhalation, ingestion, injection, skin contamination), the physical and chemical form of the contaminant, and the metabolism are known, one can decide whether to ask for a urine or fecal sample (or both), or whether to send the individual for medical collection and study of other samples (blood, tissue, etc.). It is common practice to ask at least for urine and, sometimes, fecal samples as final and reliable evidence of the presence or lack of internal exposure.

f) Making a careful examination for skin breaks of any sort. These should be checked carefully for contamination. Depending on the nature of the radiation from the contaminant, the wounds may have to be checked with more sophisticated instrumentation.

g) Collecting air samples, and carefully recording the pertinent information. Immediate measurement of air samples with portable instruments can give a good idea as to seriousness of the exposure or the continuing hazard. One must realize that the natural radioactivity of air will give beta-particle radioactivity *disintegration* rates normally ranging from 100 to 600 disintegrations per minute per cubic meter of air sampled. The beta-particle activity is normally 1.5 to 2 times as intense as the alpha-particle activity. The decay rate usually is that of radon daughters, a little less than 0.5-hour half life, but may appear to be as much as forty minutes if thoron daughters are present at the higher levels of their natural occurrence. It should be remembered that most air samplers collect aerosols at a much higher than breathing rate and with better efficiency. This should be taken into account.

h) Setting in motion the procedures for evaluating all dosimeters, bioassay samples, air samples, and smears. In all cases of radiation measurement and estimation of dose, some advance state of capability is necessary. The dosimeters should be checked for contamination. If contamination is present, it must be eliminated or its effect on the readings minimized.

i) Sending screened persons to the proper treatment station with careful, concise instructions.

II. Medical Screening

The cases which will be sent to or turned over to the medical personnel will depend somewhat on what the physician wants to see.

In general, cases in which the physician will be interested include:

1) All individuals with skin lesions of any sort whatever. It is not always possible to tell with portable instruments whether or not a wound is contaminated.

2) All individuals with serious radiation or other injuries.

3) Contaminated persons who have received significant skin dosages. The term "significant" needs defining. In practice, the plant physician is allowed to determine his own levels (usually 25 rads to 100 rads are minima).

4) Cases in which contamination is not satisfactorily removed by the decontamination team. Contamination fixed on the skin which promises, by virtue of long half life and proximity of source, to give a significant skin dose and which is not removable by ordinary methods should probably receive medical attention before the skin is injured in the decontamination procedure.

In an actual case, there will have to be some freedom for decision by medical personnel, since the way in which a physician spends his time depends very much on the number of patients to be treated, and on the severity and nature of the injuries. However, the interests of the physician can be stated and followed for small accidents which have a relatively high frequency of occurrence.

III. Screening of Materials and Equipment

Materials and equipment removed from an accident scene are screened for contamination. This work can be done without urgency, since added radiation dosage to the material is usually unimportant and since most materials are not involved with physiological, psychological and sociological life processes. In a few cases, personal effects will need to be checked for contamination under the press of people's anxieties.

IV. Screening of Emergency Workers Who Move into and out of the Accident Area

This screening is carried on in the same manner as is the screening for uninjured accident victims. It is done throughout all activities, including restoration. For the most part, it is done at a more leisurely pace; the emergency workers are usually wearing protective clothing and limiting their exposure, so that injury is very unlikely. Dosimeters are worn which can give the accumulated dose at any time.

V. What Should a Screener Know?

1) He should be familiar with the whole structure for handling emergencies which exists in his plant, and should know his own responsibilities within that plan in detail. Emergency systems usually involve capability to deal with many sizes and types of accident. The screener should know how to set the emergency plans in motion in order to get adequate coverage for whatever type of emergency he faces. Channels should exist for handling the expected classes of screened victims.

Emergency plans should include the designation of sets of technically trained and prepared persons to aid with dose evaluation, to handle medical cases, and to handle personnel decontamination problems. The specific responsibilities of such groups should be spelled out. Objectives of the whole emergency setup and each part of it should be clearly known.

2) The screener should have the general knowledge and training of a good health physics surveyor.

He should have experience and training in the handling and use of radiation and radioactivity measuring instruments. He should know what the instrument readings mean, or how to make them meaningful. He should know the limitations of the various survey meters and their capabilities. He should know how to detect and measure the various radiations within a wide range of dose rates.

He should know enough about dosimetry to know what information and samples to collect. He should be able to pick out with certainty persons who are likely to have significant exposures.

He should have some basic knowledge in nuclear science. Especially useful are knowledge of radionuclides, their properties and radiations, how radiations act with matter, how to use pertinent information in radiological health handbooks, and so on.

He should know how to handle radioactive materials without contaminating himself and especially his instruments. A contaminated instrument can be useless until decontaminated.

3) He should be familiar with dosimetry (see H. R. Fish, p. 207). At least, he should know the following:

How to get answers from common dosimeters.

How to get in touch with a few experts in a hurry.

How to determine the kind of radiation exposure involved.

To obtain and keep correct records as to location of persons exposed, time exposed in each location, radiation readings in various locations, and the time when these are taken.

What evidences of exposure to collect. He should know how to make rough estimates from these so that he can accomplish screening. He should know what information and materials to turn over to experts in dosimetry, so that they can make accurate determinations of dosage received. Evidence of exposure which leads to evaluation of dosage may be gathered and studied over periods of time ranging from minutes to weeks, depending on the type and extent of the exposure and the accuracy desired.

The following types of dosimetric measurements should be considered:

Radiation dose rates taken at the scene and considered with a map of the accident scene showing victims' locations and movements, time the exposure started and ended, the time when the readings of dose rate were taken, source information such as the decay rate of the radioisotopes involved or operating conditions of any radiation-producing machines and type and quality of the radiation. This information can lead to good dosage estimates.

Contamination surveys and air sampling data will be useful in determining the need for collection of bioassay samples or for making total body counts. Information as to the specific radioisotopes involved will be helpful in evaluating such samples and counts.

If the isotopes are unknown, samples may be collected for use in obtaining such information.

Film badges, other personal dosimeters, and foils placed on individuals can give information as to the dose received and the nature of the radiation. However, any information available about the type and hardness of the radiation, and other exposure information such as the location of the dosimeter on the body, the orientation of the body with respect to the radiation source, shielding and scatter conditions will usually be helpful in evaluating the dosimeter readings. Dosimeters should be checked for contamination, so that this information can be used in evaluating the readings. Contamination of a dosimeter can, and occasionally does, make its dosage information useless.

Results of body surveys with portable counters can be useful. Geiger counter measurements of sodium activation in the body by neutron exposure have been reported (6) as useful in obtaining rough estimates of exposure. Thyroid counts are also useful. However, in making such measurements, great care should be taken to differentiate between external contamination readings and internal radiation readings. Pre-accident calibrations of activation counts, thyroid counts, etc., are necessary to give meaning to on-site measurements.

Ion chamber measurements of skin contamination dose rates coupled with special calibrations or prepared calibration graphs (5) can give estimates of skin dosage if time of exposure and half life of the contaminants are known. If calculations have to be made, the kind and quality of the radiation should be known.

Estimates of neutron exposure can be obtained by radiochemical analysis and counting of many materials, those most commonly used being components of special criticality dosimeter systems (2, 3), blood (sodium), hair, and metallic objects. If such objects are collected, they should be carefully labeled as to location on the body or in the plant at the time of exposure, since dosage to various parts of the body and in different locations can vary considerably. Measurement of radioactive sodium in blood coupled with data from systems of threshold foils, gamma dosimeters, and indicators of body orientation can help give fairly accurate dosage estimates for mixtures of neutrons and gamma radiations. Such dosimeters and foil systems should be collected and turned over to persons prepared to evaluate them.

The results of careful measurement of radioactivity in wounds should be furnished to physicians. Such knowledge can be helpful in making medical decisions as to treatment.

4) He should be familiar with the concept of *action levels.*

Action levels are specific levels of exposure, radiation, or contamination, below which one attitude is allowed to reign and above which a different attitude prevails. For example, several action levels can exist for clothing contamination for each of many contaminants. Usually, about three or four levels are used. There is a low level below which clothing is permitted to be worn and above which decontamination is required. A second level may exist below which the individual is told to change and launder his clothing when he gets home and above which he is asked to change clothing immediately, with the laundering to be done in a facility for handling contaminated clothing. A third level may exist below which the individual's clothing is changed and laundered, but above which the clothing is disposed of as radioactive waste. Such action levels are based on the many permissible or guidance levels listed in laws and government regulations, as well as on economic and other factors. Permissible or guidance levels are usually the basis for calculation of other action levels. The action levels used in a given facility depend pretty much on the radioactive materials which are being used.

Action levels exist in two sets. The set generally in use consists of the permissible levels for chronic exposure combined with some levels calculated from these. A second set exists for civil defense purposes. Neither set has been worked out completely enough to give all the action levels necessary for emergencies. Action levels should be determined for situations which may occur. If a surveyor at the scene of an accident is faced with the necessity of setting up an action level, his service may be slowed considerably and he is likely to be quite indecisive.

A set of action levels for final, standard, and operational clearance has been worked out for Navy use (5). These include levels for skin, clothing, and work surfaces and are based on the Code of Federal Regulations, Title 10, Part 20, Federal Register, with assumed resuspension and transfer factors. They are based on the assumption of a more or less continuous duty operation. Such levels are adequate for the kinds of accidents which frequently occur, but, since they are based on an "unknown isotope*" premise, they are more restrictive than needed for some cases. Hence, similar action levels should probably be set up for your own conditions in your own emergency manual or plans. Such levels are likely to be based on the air or water maximum permissible levels legally recognized for your operation.

Probably, an additional set of action levels should be recognized, taking into account a factor for the rarity of occurrence of a really severe emergency in which hundreds of persons might suffer injuries

*It is common practice to operate using permissible levels for the most hazardous radioisotope of a type if the exact radioisotopes involved are not known.

or contamination. Most emergency plans are set up with definite limits as to the number of clothing changes and the facilities for handling accidents which are available. Furthermore, under emergency conditions there may be circumstances which make it unwise to try to detain persons with contamination spots which give rise to exposures of a fraction of a mrad or even a few mrad of beta-gamma ray emitter on their clothing, as would be required by routine action levels. On very rare occasions and under extreme emergency conditions only, it should be acceptable to release people, with proper instructions, carrying, for example, one to ten permissible body burdens of a radioisotope on their clothing.

This is a fair amount of radioactivity which, for cobalt-60, for example, would give 130 to 1,330 milliroentgens per hour at one centimeter if the whole amount were in a single spot.

Questions such as the following should be answered for your emergency preparation:

What should be the allowable levels of clothing contamination under various conditions?

At what level should clothing be seized?

What levels of contamination can be removed from clothing in the home laundry?

At what levels of external contamination should medical attention be considered?

At what levels or conditions should further screening tests be instigated?

At what levels of radiation and air contamination should a severly injured (non-radiation) person be moved?

Answers often depend on local factors.

The activities of emergency workers can be quite precise and rapid if guide lines for emergency action are known. Action levels provide such guidance.

5) He should have good knowledge of the possible types of radiation hazards in the area of his jurisdiction. This should include specific knowledge as to what radioisotopes are in use or stored in his area, and where, as well as the physical and chemical characteristics of the radioisotopes (including the chemical compounds involved) that relate to hazard potential, detection, and identification.

6) He should know about the availability and location of emergency supplies. He should have emergency access to general material stores. If his own emergency equippage is meager, channels to possible suppliers of emergency materials and services may be set up and occasionally reviewed.

7) He should know that accident victims need to be given clear, precise directions as to what to do and where to go. Emergency plans will help, but usually some judgment must be used at the scene. If there are serious injuries, a medical doctor should do the screening. Most medical emergency plans call for clearly tagging the victims, giving all the vital information possible. If a doctor is not present, first aid should be given and the patients tagged, giving as much information as possible relative to their radiation exposure and other injuries.

8) The experts who may be called on to give special service are screeners and, among them, should know the details of the various measurement methods called for. They should be able to:

a) Analyse radiochemically for any radioisotope in the bioassay samples.

b) Analyse hair, clothing, metallic objects, and other materials for neutron activation products with the aim of determining information useful in calculating neutron dose.

c) Evaluate expertly the various dosimeters including whatever criticality dosimeters may be in use.

d) Do whole-body counting if a facility is available.

e) Have enough technical competence to pull the strings of evidence together and come up with good conclusions as to what happened and what doses of radiation were received. Of course, if neutron exposures are not a possibility, the expert will not need to know (b) above, since it has value only for estimating neutron dose.

VI. Equipment List for Screening

1) Protective clothing should be available. In areas where radioactive materials are handled routinely, it is customary for all personnel to wear some sort of protective clothing, such as shoes and coveralls, continuously. In addition, gloves, respiratory protective equipment, and shoe covers should always be available. Head covers may be

useful. It should be understood that protective clothing is used only to avoid contaminating the body and personal effects with radioactive materials.

2) An assortment of portable radiation detection and measurement instruments is usually available. Capability should be on hand to measure any type and quantity of radiation that could result from a radiation accident.

3) Tags, pencils, paper, plastic bags, rope should be on hand.

4) A questionnaire and check list may be useful. A questionnaire, in some cases, cannot or should not be used, but in others, it can be helpful by presenting to persons involved in accidents some well-thought-out questions that aim at getting vital information. If the accident plans are specific, instruction sheets may be useful. These would have to fit the special case.

5) A simple decontamination kit for cleaning instruments and vital tools of the trade is useful, as is a supply of cleansing tissue.

VII. Planning for Screening

Screening is an integral part of accident handling. Hence, general plans are, in part, screening plans, except that the screener makes more detailed plans of his own designated areas of responsibility. Radiation emergency planning should include the following:

a) A survey of the installation. Mapping is useful. All sources of radiation, radioactivity and fissionable materials should be listed and studied. The types of potential accidents such as contamination, explosion, fluid leaks, etc., should be determined.

b) An estimate of the number of people involved should be made.

c) A survey of resources should be made and their usefulness relative to the accident types evaluated.

d) Objectives for emergency planning should be clearly written.

e) Responsibilities for adequate emergency planning and activity should be specifically delegated.

f) Each shift of workers should have sufficient training and organization to handle any accident or emergency condition during the initial period (1).

g) Plans should include routine reviews of emergency plans and should be aimed at keeping up interest and at improving knowledge and skills of the emergency workers.

h) Responsibility for technical capability should be designated and established.

i) Action levels should be determined.

j) Emergency materials, equipment, and instruments should be located strategically and such locations indicated in writing.

k) Planning should result in a living emergency system. A living system must continuously be supported by budgeting money, making a position for it in the organizational structure, and by relating it to real work as much as is reasonably possible.

An educational effort is a part of planning. In order to get consistent, thorough emergency action, procedural suggestions and check lists (4) as shown in Appendices II-1, II-2, II-3, and II-4 may be developed. Radiation safety workers are then asked to familiarize themselves with them and to work them into their own area plans and training procedures.

APPENDIX II-1

Special Bioassay Samples (4)

I. Special bioassay samples may be requested by Radiation Safety when the need arises. The responsibilities of a Radiation Safety requestor are listed below:

A. Notify the Radiation Safety Section Head or his authorized representative of:

1. The request (type and number of samples).
2. The reason for the request.
3. The analysis desired.
4. Special instructions (as necessary).

B. Provide the appropriate containers for urine and/or fecal samples. If necessary, instruct the person(s) submitting the samples in their proper use. If blood or sputum samples or nasal smears are required, arrangements must be made with the Health Division.

C. Instruct person(s) submitting urine or fecal samples to return the samples to the Radiation Safety requestor.

D. Prepare Form "Request for Bioassay Analysis" (see Figure II-2).

E. Immediately, upon receipt of the sample(s), transport to the bioassay laboratory, along with the Form.

REQUEST FOR BIOASSAY ANALYSIS

☐ Special
☐ Non-routine

Date of Incident:__________ Time:__________ Building:__________

Isotopes Involved:__________

Estimated Amounts: Small μc mc c mg g Other__________

Chemical Form:__________

Physical State: liquid solid gas powder solution Other__________

Names of People Involved (Include Division):__________

Nature of Incident:__________

Remarks:__________

Requested By:__________

Deliver to Bioassay Group,

FIGURE II-2.

II. *Major Incident (Working Hours)*

The bioassay sample procedures, as listed in Section I, should also be followed in the case of a major incident. In addition, bioassay samples should be requested from personnel involved and subject to the following conditions:

A. Person(s) directly involved in the area at the time of the incident.

B. Person(s) involved in subsequent activities in and about the incident area.

C. Person(s) sustaining cuts, abrasions, punctures, etc. of the skin, from material suspected or known to be contaminated.

D. Person(s) known or suspected of being downwind of the incident and prior to the determination of airborne concentrations.

These are the minimum requirements for requesting bioassay samples in the event of a major incident. This *does not* relieve any Health Physicist of the responsibility for requesting bioassay samples from personnel, for reasons other than those listed as minimal.

III. *Major Incidents (Off-Shift Hours)*

The following action should be taken by "off-shift" Radiation

Safety personnel in the event of any incident:

A. Initiate the bioassay sample procedures as outlined in Sections I and II.

B. Instruct person(s) submitting urine or fecal samples to return the samples to a specific location.

C. Provide Radiation Safety personnel, at the specified delivery point, with pertinent data.

APPENDIX II-2

Radiation Safety Control Center Procedure Check (4)

The procedures listed herein should be considered as a guide or aid in handling incident situations. The order of consideration of the individual items listed should be determined to suit the particular incident.

Personnel

1. Are all personnel involved at incident site accounted for?
2. Have personnel been surveyed?
   a) Are personnel segregated as to contamination and/or induced activity levels?
   b) Injuries noted?
   c) Has decontamination been attempted and results noted?
   d) Were personnel monitoring devices collected?
   e) Have all pertinent data pertaining to personnel been remanded to Health Services?
3. Have personnel downwind of the incident been notified?
4. Have the proper bioassay procedures been initiated?
   a) Samples from persons involved?
   b) Samples from persons injured with contamination or suspect contaminated material?
   c) Persons downwind?
   d) Persons subsequently involved?
   e) Have sample kits been distributed?
   f) Have sample kits been returned?
   g) Have data been submitted to bioassay?
   h) Have results been received?
   i) Have results been reported to pertinent authority?
5. Have measures been instituted to control ingress and egress of personnel into hazard area?

a) Guards been notified?
b) Site Administration notified?
c) Barriers erected?

6. Have measures been instituted to protect personnel on re-entry?
   a) Protective clothing and shoe covers.
   b) Respiratory equipment.
   c) Knowledge of radiation hazard.
   d) Knowledge of other hazards.

Evaluation

1. Have surveys been made outside of the control area?
   a) Radiological Assistance Team utilized?
   b) Air samples taken downwind?
   c) Peripheral surveys made?
   d) Surveys made of vehicles and/or equipment used in incident?
   e) Have "continuous operation" instruments been checked for data?
   f) Personnel monitor device results been recorded?
2. Have surveys been made of the incident area?
   a) Contamination levels?
   b) Background levels?
   c) Air samples taken and recorded?
   d) Accident dosimeters retrieved?
3. Have contacts been initiated with personnel familiar with the incident facility?
   a) Personnel involved, if possible?
   b) Plant Services for that area?
   c) Plant Engineering.
   d) Others.

Instrumentation and Equipment

1. Has sufficient instrumentation been acquired?
   a) Portable.
   b) Alternating current counters.
   c) Analyzers.
   d) Air samplers (particulate and gas).
   e) Portable alternating current generators (when needed).
2. Is an instrument repairman on hand for limited repair work?

Protective Apparel

Has sufficient apparel been procured?

a) Coveralls.
b) Underclothing.
c) Shoe covers.
d) Gloves.

Respiratory Devices

Is there a supply of proper respirators to meet the need?

a) Scott Air Paks.
b) Supplied-air suits.
c) Assault Masks and cannisters.
d) Dust respirators.
e) Other.

Control

1. Have measures been instituted to contain the incident?
   a) Fire extinguishers.
   b) Ventilation shutdown (when needed).
   c) Cause area isolated.
   d) Utilities secured.
   e) Hazard area isolated.
   f) Shoe cover change areas and survey points set up.
2. Have measures been taken to insure against recurrence of incident?
   a) Discussion with personnel familiar with incident apparatus.
   b) Assistance in developing methods of neutralization of incident apparatus.

Transportation

Are there sufficient vehicles on hand?

a) General transportation.
b) Survey vehicles.
c) Decontamination vehicles (bulldozers, road graders, tankers, etc.).
d) Other.

Communications

Have communications been established?

a) Telephone.

b) Mobile radio.
c) Portable radio.
d) Laboratory radio.

Plant and Facilities (Immediate)

Have measures been taken to reduce the loss or damage to plant equipment?

a) Secure utilities.
b) Neutralize destructive conditions (fires, acids, water, etc.).

Plant and Facilities (Restoration)

Have measures been taken to restore facilities?

a) Assist in developing techniques with proper authorities.
b) Consult with Reclamation Services (decontamination).

Security

Have proper measures been taken to safeguard security items and/or areas?

Reporting

Is a running log of events and data being compiled?

a) Survey of personnel.
b) Personnel exposures.
c) Survey of periphery.
d) Survey immediate area.
e) Bioassay results.
f) Manpower used.
g) Instrumentation and equipment used.
h) Progress of control.
i) Control measures taken.

Have the Radiation Safety activities been reported to proper authority?

a) Laboratory Director or authorized representative.
b) Technical Services Manager.
c) Laboratory Control Center.
d) Other.

APPENDIX II-3

Guide for Radiation Safety Control Center Supervisors (4)

The purpose of this guide is to establish procedures as a basis for the operation of Radiation Safety Control Centers (R.S.C.C.).

In cases involving major incidents, the Control Center supervisor will be the Radiation Safety Section Head or his authorized representative.

General Objectives of Radiation Safety in their order of concern:

1. Personnel immediately involved.
2. Personnel indirectly involved (downwind, etc.).
3. Personnel subsequently involved (re-entry personnel).
4. Control of incident (isolation).
5. Control of incident recurrence.
6. The reporting of preliminary Health Physics technical information.
7. Plant and facilities immediate.
8. Plant and facilities restoration.
9. Security (when needed).

The duties of the Radiation Safety Control Center supervisor are as follows:

1. Select site to be used as the Control Center.
   a) Select R.S.C.C. as close to incident site as is practicable.
   b) R.S.C.C. should have facilities for the operation and limited repair of instrumentation.
   c) Facilities should be available for the decontamination of personnel and instrumentation.
   d) Communication facilities should be at hand or readily installed.
2. Acquire sufficient manpower to meet the need.
   a) List of Radiation Safety personnel contacts both off and on shift.
3. Evaluate situation.
4. Develop method(s) for control of the situation.
5. Procure sufficient instrumentation and equipment as needed.
6. Assignment of duties of Radiation Safety personnel.
7. Maintain liaison with other authorities.
8. Maintain a running log of all events and information.
9. Location of and contacts for pertinent facilities, items and equipment (list location and phone number for regular hours and off-shift hours for the following):
   Environmental monitoring services.

Bioassay services.
Carpenter shop.
Communications.
Mobile air compressors (for air-supplied suits).
Active waste containers, dry and liquid.
Trash containers.
Shielded containers.
Decontamination equipment, general, heavy duty, contractors.
Engineering drawings of site and buildings.
Electricians.
Mobile electric generators.
Instruments (general survey, analyzers, whole-body counters, criticality dosimeter processors, personal dosimetry, instrument repair, electric stock).
Locksmith.
Meteorology.
Heavy-duty movers (riggers).
Protective apparel (coveralls, shoe covers, gloves, shoes, caps, toe rubbers—stockrooms, emergency supplies, regular supplies).
Radiochemical analysis.
Radiological assistance team.
Respiratory protective supplies (supplied-air paks and supplies, supplied-air suits, assault masks and cannisters, dust respirators).
Security personnel (police, plant guards).
Transportation (passenger, ambulances, heavy-duty vehicles, vehicle repair).
Utilities (electrical distribution, steam, water, gas, ventilation).

APPENDIX II-4

Questionnaire: Personal Statement Concerning Incident*

Name____________________ Dosimeter No.__________
Date of incident____________________ Time__________AM PM
Supervisor____________________
Job assignment____________________
Where were you at the time of the incident?____________________
Show on map. (If maps are used, prepare in advance.)

*This questionnaire is a reworked model of that appearing in Reference (1).

How did you recognize or how were you informed of the emergency?__________

____

How soon did you leave your location after knowing of emergency?__________

____

What action did you take at the time of the incident if you did not leave immediately? (Specify particularly any actions to control emergency.)__________

____

How did you leave the area? Walk?__________ Run?__________

Mark the route on map.

Did you see, hear, feel, or smell anything unusual? Describe__________

____

Do you know where any of your co-workers were or what they were doing at the time of the incident? (Indicate location on map.)__________

____

Do you know the location of the accidental event? (Indicate on map.)__________

____

Name all the other persons you know were in the building (area).__________

____

Do you have other comments?__________

REFERENCES

1. Bahler, K. W., Rupp, A. F., Lafferty, R. H., Wachter, J. W., and O'Rourke, L. S.: *Prevention and Handling of Radiation Emergencies.* Oak Ridge Gaseous Diffusion Plant, Report K-1436, Dec. 1959.
2. Hoy, J. E.: *An Emergency Neutron Dosimeter.* E. I. duPont de Nemours and Co., Savannah River Laboratory, Report DP-472, Sept. 1960.
3. Hurst, G. S., and Ritchie, R. H.: *Radiation Accidents: Dosimetric Aspects of Neutron and Gamma-Ray Exposures.* Oak Ridge National Laboratory, Report ORNL-2748 Part A, 1959.
4. Smith, W. H., Dyer, N. C., and Lonergan, G. T.: Unpublished internal reports reproduced with minor changes. Argonne National Laboratory, Argonne, Illinois.
5. Sulit, R. A., Leahy, E. J., and Baietti, A. L.: *Principles of Radiation and Contamination Control.* U.S. Naval Radiological Defense Laboratory, Report NAVSHIPS 250-341-3, Vol. III, 195?.
6. Wilson, R. H.: *A Method for Immediate Detection of High Level Neutron Exposure by Measurement of Sodium-24 in Humans.* Hanford Atomic Products Operation, Report HW-73891 (Rev), July 31, 1962.

EMERGENCY BIOASSAY METHODS

JACOB SEDLET

*Argonne National Laboratory**
Argonne, Illinois

In the present context, bioassay refers to the determination of above-normal amounts of radioactive materials inside the body by whatever means are appropriate. In emergencies, results should be obtained within minutes or hours. High sensitivity is not required, since one has the advantage, when measurements are made early, that the activity to be detected is greatest. In this discussion, it is assumed that the detection of an intake equivalent to the smallest continuous maximum permissible body burden (MPBB) specified by the International Commission on Radiological Protection (7) is adequate.

I. Whole-body Counting

The first method which should be considered in an emergency is whole-body, or *in vivo,* counting. Perhaps little need be said about whole-body counters, not only because of their limited availability, but also because laboratories which have calibrated whole-body counting facilities are familiar with their function and applicability. However, if the situation warrants their use, most existing facilities would probably be available for counting contaminated individuals from laboratories which do not have such equipment. Whole-body counting has the advantages of speed, accuracy, and good sensitivity. Counting times are short, less than thirty minutes, and a direct measurement of the desired quantity, the body radioactivity, is obtained.

There are two principal limitations. First, the radiation obviously must leave the body, restricting the method to nuclides that emit moderately energetic gamma or x-rays, or to energetic beta-ray emitters (in which case the bremsstrahlung is counted). In addition,

*Operated by The University of Chicago for the U.S. Atomic Energy Commission.

a single measurement probably will not distinguish between active material in the body and that on the skin and hair.

Four types of detectors are now in use: sodium iodide crystals (1, 6, 12, 13, 14, 15), liquid scintillators (1, 2, 6, 14), plastic scintillators (3), and gas-filled proportional counters (8). The sodium iodide crystal is the most common and generally applicable detector, although each type has advantages for certain purposes. Sodium iodide gives the best energy resolution (except for very low-energy radiation, i.e., less than about 25 kev) and permits one to determine activity distributions in the body, while liquid and plastic scintillators are sufficiently inexpensive to permit one to surround most of the body with detector and consequently to obtain high counting efficiencies. Proportional counters are useful for x-rays and low-energy gamma rays since they have better resolution and backgrounds for such radiations than other detectors. It is worth noting that elaborate shielding ("iron rooms") and very large detectors are not necessary for adequate whole-body counting of most nuclides (17, 22, 23).

A whole-body counter can be improvised for many conceivable emergency situations by using an available sodium iodide crystal, with shielding composed of lead bricks, iron plates, or thick concrete walls or floors in the manner of the Hanford "shadow shield" (17, 22). It is important to shield the crystal; in addition, some shielding against external gamma radiation can be provided. If gamma-ray spectrometry is not required, counting can be done with a conventional pulse height discriminator and scaler. At sufficiently high activity levels, spectrometry can be performed with a single-channel rather than a multichannel analyzer. The problem of calibrating a hastily improvised arrangement remains.

Table II-1 lists some common nuclides which can be detected in amounts less than the continuous MPBB by whole-body counting for less than one hour. The two beta particle emitters are best determined by counting the bremsstrahlung with a thin sodium iodide crystal (10, 11, 18, 19). Thorium-232 must be determined by counting its decay products; therefore, it is more difficult to estimate after accidental intake than the other nuclides. Plutonium-239 can be detected in wounds with good sensitivity (approximately 10^{-4} μc) by counting the x-rays emitted by its uranium daughter, using a thin crystal scintillator (21). Thin crystals and gas-filled counters will probably give adequate sensitivity for plutonium in the lung, but not in the skeleton (8, 20). Similarly, in the lung, the determination of less than the MPBB of uranium with any enrichment is feasible (4). Sufficiently sensitive skeleton determinations, however, may be limited to highly enriched uranium.

II. Blood and Elimination Analyses

If *in vivo* counting is not available or appropriate, it will be necessary to determine the body content from the elimination rate or the blood concentrations of the nuclide. This requires a knowledge of the relation between these quantities which is, unfortunately, difficult to obtain for a real situation. However, large numbers of samples can be processed rapidly and external contamination is not an important problem. Urine and fecal samples are used to measure elimination rates. Breath can be sampled for radioactive gases. Blood should be at least as useful as urine, but has not been employed as frequently, perhaps because results are difficult to interpret and samples are difficult to obtain. If the nuclides emit electromagnetic radiation in sufficient abundance, the samples should be counted with a sodium iodide crystal or other gamma or x-ray detector since no sample preparation is involved.

Analyzers are useful and convenient, but not necessary unless unknown nuclides are involved. If alpha or beta particle activity must be detected, simple and rapid chemical separations are indicated. Rapid chemical methods (1-2 hours) are probably limited to blood volumes less than 10-15 ml and urine volumes less than about 100 ml. The chemical analysis of a fecal sample will require perhaps six additional hours, and a twenty-four-hour urine sample perhaps two to three additional hours. Many nuclides, especially when inhaled in a form not readily soluble in biological fluids, are eliminated primarily in the feces, while, in some situations, only the fraction contained in the blood and urine is important in terms of long-term body deposition. In general, all types of samples should be collected, even if the analysis of fecal samples must be delayed. It should be pointed out that, although speed is important, it is possible to collect a sample too soon after exposure, before the maximum concentration is reached in the blood or excreta.

Table II-2 gives the detectable amounts of a number of nuclides by excretion analyses that can be completed in about one hour. The values were determined for the following conditions: Samples and backgrounds are counted for fifteen minutes; the minimum detectable amount is then taken as three times the standard deviation of a fifteen-minute background. Direct counting of tritium and carbon-14 is done with 0.5 ml of sample in a lead-shielded liquid scintillation counter, with two cooled phototubes recording coincident pulses. Direct counting of the other nuclides is done with a solid 4 in. x 4 in. lead-shielded sodium iodide scintillator crystal using 250 ml of urine (about one-sixth of a daily output) or an entire fecal sample. Alpha and beta particle counting of separated activity is performed in a 2π gas-flow counter, two inches in diameter, and with alpha and beta particle backgrounds of 0.1 and fifty counts per minute, respectively. The separations are performed on 50 ml of urine (about one-thirtieth of a daily output). There are several ways of improving the sensitivity, some requiring additional time. The efficiency of gamma-ray counting can be increased by evaporating urine samples to provide better geometry, or by using two opposed crystals or a well crystal. Chemical separations can be performed on larger samples. This will improve the sensitivity in proportion to the increase in sample size. An increase in counting time or decrease in background improves the sensitivity by the square root of the change.

The sensitivity of blood analysis by chemical separation would be similar, per sample, as for urine. That is, the minimum detectable amount would be one-thirtieth of the values in Table II-2. The sensitivity by direct counting would be the same as given in Table II-2 for the same sample size. Since smaller samples would be taken, the actual sensitivity would be improved by the improvement in geometry.

It must still be determined whether the sensitivities provided by these types of analyses are sufficient for detecting potentially toxic amounts. The behavior of radioactive materials in the body shortly after their accidental intake is difficult to ascertain, and is certainly variable. However, by any criteria, if the samples are collected during the first day or two after intake, the minimum detectable amounts in Table II-2 are adequate for all nuclides except possibly for the bone seekers (calcium, strontium, radium, thorium, plutonium, and americium). The bone seekers present a separate problem, and the adequacy of the values given depends on the parameters chosen to describe their retention and elimination. This is illustrated for plutonium-239 in Table II-3.

Using an exponential model and the biological half lives given by the International Commission on Radiological Protection (7), a sensitivity of 9 pc/day (picocurie per day) is satisfactory for inhalation exposures, but not for injections. However, the half life for bone given by the Commission is conservative when applied to times soon after deposition. It appears that the elimination of bone seekers can be described best by a power function (9, 16). In this case, the sensitivity of detection soon after injection or bone deposition is adequate, but the sensitivity for inhalation exposures must be improved by a factor of about ten. This can be done, as was indicated previously, and will add one to three hours to the time required for analysis.

III. Chemical Methods

Table II-4 gives some rapid chemical methods for analysis of urine samples, which can be completed in about one hour if urine volumes less than 100 ml are used. These methods can be used for much larger urine samples and for fecal samples, but several additional hours will be required to concentrate or ash and dissolve the specimens. Blood samples can be analyzed by the same methods after the organic matter has first been oxidized with, for example, nitric acid and hydrogen peroxide. Ten ml of blood can be oxidized in about one hour.

All of these methods use precipitation or solvent extraction separations, since such separations can be done rapidly. Ion exchange separations generally require more time, but it is possible that they could be adapted for emergency use. When chemical separations are performed on unashed (or raw) urine, the chemical nature of the excreted radionuclides can cause difficulties. Some elements can be excreted in forms which do not undergo the expected reactions, probably because they are complexed or colloidal. The excreted forms can sometimes be returned to their more simple ionic forms by acidifying and heating the urine. This problem can only be studied with urine containing naturally excreted nuclides, and such material is not readily available.

Uranium in urine is best determined by measuring its fluorescence in a sodium fluoride matrix. The method can detect, in less than thirty minutes, about three pc of normal uranium and 300 pc of enriched uranium in 1500 ml. This sensitivity is adequate for emergencies.

IV. Summary

Emergency bioassay measurements should be performed by *in vivo* counting if this method is applicable and available. Estimates of internal contamination can readily be made by analyzing blood and elimination samples. Chemical methods are available for such analyses when direct counting of the sample cannot be done. However, the analysis of such samples is easier than the interpretation of the results in terms of body burden.

TABLE II-1

COMMON NUCLIDES WHICH CAN BE DETERMINED IN AMOUNTS LESS THAN THE CONTINUOUS MAXIMUM PERMISSIBLE BODY BURDEN BY WHOLE-BODY COUNTING

P^{32}	Many Rare Earth Fission Products
Cr^{51}	Ir^{192}
Mn^{54}	Hg^{203}
Fe^{59}	Ra^{226}
Zn^{65}	(Th^{232})
Sr^{90}-Y^{90}	(Pu^{239})
Zr^{95}-Nb^{95}	(U-natural)
Ru^{106}	(U-enriched)
$Te^{127m,129m}$	Am^{241}
I^{131}	
Cs^{137}	

TABLE II-2

MINIMUM AMOUNTS DETECTABLE BY EXCRETION ANALYSIS

	Direct Counting		*Chemical Separation*
	Urine	*Feces*	*Urine*
Nuclide	*(pc/1500 ml)*	*(pc/sample)*	*(pc/1500 ml)*
H^3 (as water)	6.7×10^4	—	—
C^{14}	1.8×10^4	—	—
P^{32}, Sr^{90}	—	—	150

S^{35}, Ca^{45}, Tc^{99}, Pm^{147}	—	—	200
Fe^{59}	200	40	—
Co^{60}	100	20	—
Zn^{65}	180	35	—
Zr^{95}, Nb^{95}	250	50	—
Ru^{106}	125	25	—
Te^{127m}	500	100	—
I^{131}	150	30	—
Cs^{137}	300	60	—
Ce^{144}	450	90	—
Ra^{226}	950	190	9
Actinide Alpha Particle Emitters	—	—	9
Am^{241}	300	60	9

TABLE II-3

URINARY EXCRETION FROM 0.04 μc PLUTONIUM AFTER ONE DAY (IN PICOCURIES PER DAY)

Exponential Function (7)		*Power Function (5, 9)*	
Bone	*Lung*	*Bone*	*Lung*
0.38	23	70	ca. 1

TABLE II-4

CHEMICAL METHODS FOR EMERGENCY BIOASSAY ANALYSES

Element	*Procedure*
Calcium, Barium, Strontium, Rare Earths	Precipitate calcium oxalate or phosphate from alkaline solution. Carriers may be used.
Barium, Radium, Sulfur	Precipitate barium sulfate from acid solution. Use barium carrier for barium and radium.
Americium, Curium, Plutonium, Thorium, Promethium and other Rare Earths	Precipitate rare earth fluoride from acid solution.
Phosphorus	Precipitate calcium phosphate.
Technetium	Precipitate copper sulfide from acid solution.
Uranium, Plutonium, Thorium	Extract with solution of organic phosphate ester (diethylhexyl phosphate, etc.). Evaporate organic solution to dryness for counting.

REFERENCES

1. Allsopp, C. B., ed.: The Measurement of Body Radioactivity. *Brit. J. Radiol.*, Suppl. No. 7, 1957.

2. Anderson, E. C., Schuch, R. I., Perrings, J. L., and Langham, W. H.: The Los Alamos Human Counter. *Nucleonics, 14*:No. 1, 26-29, 1956.

3. Burch, P. R. J., Hughes, D., Iinuma, T. A., Overton, T. R., and Appleby, D. B.: The Construction and Performance of a Three-Unit Plastic Scintillator Whole-Body Counter, in *Whole-Body Counting.* Proc. of IAEA Scientific Meeting, June 12-16, 1961, Int. Atomic Energy Agency, Vienna, 1962, pp. 59-69.

4. Colfield, R. E.: *In vivo* Gamma Counting as a Measurement of Uranium in the Human Lung. *Health Physics, 2*:269-287, 1960.

5. Healy, J. W.: Estimation of Plutonium Lung Burdens by Urinanalyses. *Am. Ind. Hyg. Assoc. Quarterly, 18*:261-266, 1957.

6. *Whole-Body Counting.* Proc. of IAEA Scientific Meeting, June 12-16, 1961, Int. Atomic Energy Agency, Vienna, 1962.

7. Committee II on Permissible Dose for Internal Radiation, International Commission on Radiological Protection (1959). *Health Physics, 3*:1-380, 1960.

8. Kiefer, H., and Maushart, R.: Determination of Plutonium-239 Body Burden using Gamma Spectrometry with Proportional Counters, in *Whole-Body Counting.* Proc. of IAEA Scientific Meeting, June 12-16, 1961, Int. Atomic Energy Agency, Vienna, pp. 289-293, 1962.

9. Langham, W. H., Bassett, S. H., Harris, P. S., and Carter, R. E.: Los Alamos Scientific Laboratory, Report LA 1151, 1950.

10. Liden, K.: The Determination of Sr^{90} and other Beta Emitters in Human Beings from External Measurements of the Bremsstrahlung. *Proc. 2nd U.N. Int. Conf. PUAE,* Geneva, *23*:133-139, 1958.

11. Liden, K., and McCall, R. C.: Low-Energy-Photon Detectors for Whole-Body Counting, in *Whole-Body Counting.* Proc. of IAEA Scientific Meeting, June 12-16, 1961, Int. Atomic Energy Agency, Vienna, pp. 145-166, 1962.

12. Marinelli, L. D., Miller, C. E., Gustafson, P. F., and Rowland, R. E.: The Quantitative Determination of Gamma-Ray Emitting Elements in Living Persons. *Am. J. Roentgenol., Radium Therapy and Nucl. Med., 73*:661-671, 1955.

13. Marinelli, L. D., Miller, C. E., Rowland, R. E., and Rose, J. E.: Measurement *in vivo* of Radium Gamma-Ray Activities Lower than K^{40} Levels Existing in the Human Body. *Radiology, 64*:116, 1955.

14. Meneely, G. R., ed.: *Radioactivity in Man.* Charles C Thomas, Publisher, Springfield, 1961.

15. Miller, C. E.: Low-intensity Spectrometry of the Gamma Radiation Emitted by Human Beings. *Proc. 2nd U.N. Int. Conf., PUAE,* Geneva, *23*:113-122, 1958.

16. Norris, W. P., Tyler, S. A., and Brues, A. M.: Retention of Radioactive Bone Seekers. *Science, 128*:456-62, 1958.

17. Palmer, H. E., in Gamertsfelder, C. C., and Green, J. K., ed.: Hanford Atomic Products Operation, Report HW-77609, 2.1-2.15, 1963.
18. Palmer, H. E., in Gamertsfelder, C. C., and Green, J. K., ed.: Hanford Atomic Products Operation, Report HW-77609, 2.22-2.24, 1963.
19. Palmer, H. E.: Detection of P^{32} *in vivo*. *Radiology, 78*:115, 1962.
20. Roesch, W. C., and Palmer, H. E.: Detection of Plutonium *in vivo* By Whole-Body Counting. *Health Physics, 8*:773-776, 1962.
21. Roesch, W. E., and Baum, J. W.: Detection of Plutonium in Wounds. *Proc. 2nd U.N. Int. Conf., PUAE,* Geneva, *23*:142-143, 1958.
22. Roesch, W. C., and Palmer, H. E., in Junkins, R. L., and Ashbrook, P. F., ed.: Hanford Atomic Products Operation, Report HW-70050, pp. 47-50, 1961.
23. Royster, G. W., Jr., and Fish, B. R.: E. I. duPont de Nemours and Co., Savannah River Laboratory, Report DP-831, pp. 46-57, 1962.

DISCUSSION

Dr. H. Cember (University of Cincinnati): I have a question for Dr. Oken. I frequently have noticed in the past situations in which, while personnel have been under considerable stress—this may be in a near-emergency or a "hot" operation—you come to some point at which the level of stress is too high and the person's ability to do his job safely is relatively decreased. How can we identify in advance these people who are prone to such stress, and how, on the spot, in a national emergency or in a "hot" operation, can we look for something in these people which tells us that they are under some unusually large amount of stress?

Dr. D. Oken: I don't know how well we can predict the people who will have unusually severe reactions. As I mentioned, I think we can do this a little bit, but I think military experience indicated that a great many people were turned down in certain phases of military selection on psychiatric grounds, and later on, when the need for manpower got greater, they were inducted and performed admirably, even in very difficult combat situations. So, I think our screening in this sense is not so grave. If there is severe and repeated psychiatric breakdown, sure, it becomes easy.

I think the question really comes down partly to the issue of training, as I mentioned, and partly to the area of observation. If you get somebody who does, for example, behave in an unrealistic way, does seem to deny danger, behaving with carelessness, I think it behooves you to bring this person in and talk with him and evaluate him in a somewhat more intensive and more traditional clinically psychiatric kind of way.

This is why I pointed out that I think the person who is very reliable and who, after always coming on time, begins to be late three or four times within the space of a few weeks, for example, or begins to behave in a perhaps subtle but obviously tipoff manner should be seen; and the stress, of course, may be the radiation work but may be due to a mother-in-law or some other problem.

I think it is really a question of good observation more than anything else, and then having someone around who can deal with the situation.

Dr. K. W. Newman (Turko Products, California): I'd like to direct this to Mr. Voss. His use of the example of potential spread of contamination during shipment on common carriers, I think, is a poor choice, specifically where he mentioned cobalt-60. There are several reasons for this being a poor choice, and one reason is that all such shipments must be in Interstate Commerce Commission or Bureau of Explosives approved shipping containers, able to withstand shock and fire. Secondly, even if there were damage to the container, the steel container is supposed to hold the lead even during fire. Therefore, cobalt-60 in any fire which could reach a common carrier would not probably be involved in a contaminating occurrence.

Mr. M. D. Voss: I presume that is a question, so I'll answer it. I chose that example specifically. It was presented as a real case of an unclear situation with regard to authority. I did not want to get hung with a 10,000 curie shipment loss some place, and we tried to write into the specifications who was responsible from that standpoint. Now, you are right. All of these regulations and everything are fine, except that we cannot use that cobalt at the present time. It is in our facility and it is contaminated on the outside. The inside of the container was contaminated. Everything else was just fine. But this could have spread.

I'm a little more inclined to believe that, if anything can happen, it will happen, in spite of all these things.

Dr. A. A. Spritzer (University of Pittsburgh): I just want to comment on Mr. Pingel's remarks about the cases physicians should see. He implied that the physician should determine whom he wants to see, or else that cases should be sent to the physician on the basis of some dose estimate received by the victim. I just wanted to point out that in my experience, when an accident has occurred, initially there has been a tendency both on the part of the patient and the surveying health physicist to underestimate the dose appreciably, and this is understandable. Then, when the medical department has entered into the case and estimates are formally asked from the health physics department as to exposure doses, again understandably, these have been overestimated, so that very frequently in an accident situation the physician, at least for the first few days, is left in the position of estimating exposure on the basis of biologic response rather than on physical dosimetry estimates. This being the case, then, it might be well to consider in your procedures a medical survey of all those people potentially exposed, above some minimum level, because very frequently an adverse biologic response causes the health physicist to go back and recalculate his dose.

Mr. J. H. Pingel: I have no comments. I think that is a very good suggestion.

Member: For persons who are exposed to radiation unknowingly, what types of bioassays should be taken, and what is their value in determining the injury to the person?

Dr. J. Sedlet: I believe in industrial radiography this is external exposure in which the source of radiation is intact. Is that right?

Member: That's correct.

Dr. J. Sedlet: Then bioassay procedures would not be indicated, obviously, if he has not taken any radioactive materials internally. It is a problem in dose determination by an external source or sources. If the radiation dose is severe enough, there are changes that the clinical laboratory can observe, and blood count or some other clinical findings might establish the radiation dose.

Mr. T. Fields (Health Physics Associates, Highland Park, Illinois): Along the same lines, what about those industrial radiographers who perhaps get a ruptured or leaking sealed source? What advice would you give on doing bioassays?

Dr. J. Sedlet: If there is a reasonably good chance that the person could have taken some of this material into his body, the obvious bioassay procedure would be to examine his excretions for the isotope that is used. What samples should be analyzed and by what method depends upon what the source is.

Mr. A. J. Solari (University of Michigan): This question is directed to Mr. Milo Voss. If I understood you right, you said there could be an action level at which you would abandon a victim, or evacuate private property. Could you give me some idea of what levels you were talking about in abandoning a victim or abandoning private property?

Mr. M. D. Voss: I don't want to give you an answer in numbers for that. The U.S. Atomic Energy Commission recently distributed a memorandum for comment, and I was considerably disturbed at the memo because it did everything but come out and face the fact that under certain circumstances, if you do set a level at which you will not risk your personnel, then you must remember that your dosimetry estimates can still be in error. The measured exposure rate may be 500 R/hour at one point and actual exposure rate be 10,000 R/hour at the point where you have to go. If you haven't established administrative control at the time, people may go in to rescue at considerable risk, but if you have made an evaluation in a hurry and the rescuer is obviously going to get 1,000 R (a nearly certain lethal dose) in getting somebody out, I would say that it is pretty risky and the person who was trapped or disabled in that radiation field was probably done already. I think you can quibble about fine points below that.

Dr. D. Oken: I am delighted that that question was asked. It is a very shocking statement, which is why I think the question really came up. I don't feel competent to answer it, obviously, although I assume there would be such a situation, and the reason I want to comment is that it seems to me it is important that someone did bring up this question and that we begin to think about this kind of thing, because if we decide it is too horrible to think about—and it certainly does violate our traditional ways of thinking; we are very oriented toward saving human beings at whatever cost, even the cost of other human beings—if we don't face it, this is defensive denial. If you are suddenly faced with a rescue or abandon situation, you're not likely to know what to do. If you think about it in advance, I think you can deal with your own feelings about it and then work out procedures.

Chapter III

MEDICAL RESTORATION OF PERSONNEL

DECONTAMINATION OF UNINJURED PERSONNEL

R. H. BURR AND M. G. MASON

Health and Safety Department, Uranium Division
Mallinckrodt Chemical Works
St. Charles, Missouri

THE DECONTAMINATION of uninjured personnel is not a simple application of the techniques of good personal hygiene or the routine implementation of special cleaning techniques involving prescribed chemical cleansing agents. It is, in fact, a subject which can, and often does, involve a complex and diverse spectrum of problems. Basically, the need in decontamination of uninjured personnel is for the removal of deposited radioactive material from the person's clothing and body. The purpose of decontamination is twofold:

1) To prevent the deposited radioactive material from being taken internally by the individual concerned through inhalation, ingestion, or absorption through the intact skin.

2) To remove any external radiation source from the body of the individual.

The decontamination effort can also supply pertinent information concerning the potential exposure of the individual to the radioactive material. A knowledgeable analysis of the type and quantities of radioactive material removed from the contaminated person or his clothing (provided the materials removed during decontamination are collected) may provide the only data upon which to premise an estimate of the internal and external radiation exposure to which the individual was subjected.

Decontamination of personnel serves an additional purpose, not related directly to the individual's welfare, but rather to the control and handling of the radiological emergency situation itself. Decontamination of each affected individual is a fundamental requirement for the prevention and control of the spread of radioactive contamination to other areas and to other persons.

Practically speaking, the methods employed in the handling of personnel decontamination play an important role in a well-managed plant processing radioactive materials. In the case of a radiological accident or emergency occurring away from the plant premises, particularly in public areas, the assistance rendered and the skill with which it is employed, as well as the success achieved in implementing decontamination techniques may be most important for the successful conclusion of the radiological emergency situation.

Personnel decontamination problems have been and are being handled successfully every day in various plant facilities handling, storing, and processing radioactive material. These daily problems vary in the nature and the degree of the decontamination problem, as personnel exposure problems range from those arising in operations involving a single individual working with tracer amounts of a radioisotope, to those with many persons working in large production facilities in which tons of radioactive materials are being processed daily.

In these plants, effective personnel decontamination programs are the result of skilled preplanning, thorough training of personnel, foresight in defining the need for equipment and facilities and, in many cases, the actual designing of decontamination equipment and facilities.

Preplanning and foresight in each case involve an evaluation based upon experience and a knowledgeable appraisal of the extent of the potential decontamination problem. The latter is achieved through an adequate communication system providing up-to-date and accurate information concerning plant processes, type and quantities of radioactive materials employed, production schedules, manpower usage, etc. Planned investigations involving actual measurement of personnel contamination and subsequent determinations of decontamination factors are used, in addition, to provide supplemental information. The product of such efforts can result in a personnel decontamination program which effectively answers the basic needs already described, and does so not only in day-to-day operations which may result in contamination of personnel, but also during plant radiological emergencies or other similar accident situations.

Preplanning to handle the personnel decontamination aspect of a radiological emergency includes the training of personnel in radiation monitoring techniques, in the use of protective equipment and clothing, and in the actual implementation of techniques for effective decontamination including methods, equipment, and facilities to be used. Preplanning also includes analysis and preparation in advance to cope with types of accidents of varying degrees of seriousness such as collisions or wrecks involving vehicles carrying large amounts of radioactive material, high-level fallout from atomic warfare, and accidents leading to the release of radiation or radioactive material from reactors or nuclear material processing plants.

Implicit throughout the preplanning step, and fundamental during actual radiological emergencies, is the coordination of decontamination efforts with those of other team efforts brought into play as methods of action are devised in advance, and as action is taken to cope with all aspects of the emergency circumstances. The decontamination team effort can be accomplished effectively only if complete knowledge of the situation is available. Conversely, the radiological emergency team's effort cannot be successful without the knowledge available from and the services rendered by the decontamination group.

Recognition must also be given to the significant fact that the scope of the particular emergency situation can be widely and rapidly expanded to even more serious consequences if the procedures for the decontamination of uninjured personnel are not brought into immediate operation. This is particularly true in a radiation incident which occurs in a populated area and which involves large numbers of uninjured persons.

The final component in preplanning the decontamination effort is the development of the basic plan of action. The plan must be thorough in detail, and yet provide flexibility in application.

In general, any plan of action for the decontamination of uninjured persons in a radiological emergency accident should include:

1) A plan to set up and operate a monitoring station.

2) A plan to provide for and operate a decontamination facility. This phase of the plan must include techniques for improvisation of

such a facility in the field, and provide for such additional monitoring capabilities as may be needed.

3) A plan to control personnel at the site of the incident to insure that all persons pass through the monitoring and, if need be, the decontamination stations.

The monitoring facility should be equipped with portable radiation instruments permitting detection and measurement of alpha, beta, and gamma radiations. The facility should be further equipped with items such as disposable tissues, filter paper, swabs, cotton, etc., for use in taking wipes from various parts of the bodies of contaminated persons and their clothes. Provision should be made for the storage and retention of such samples for future study.

The decontamination facility should include a station at which a person can remove his clothing. Facilities should be provided for collection of this clothing, and for its storage and retention for further study. A suitable technique for accomplishing this task is the placing of a properly sized sheet of plastic upon which the contaminated person can step. The person can then carefully take off his clothing and remove his shoes and socks directly onto this sheet. The plastic sheet can then be easily and safely folded, starting from the corners, to provide a self-contained package. The use of an outside envelope, bag, or container to hold the folded sheet is preferred particularly for identification and subsequent retention purposes. The contaminated clothing should not be disposed of until later study has determined the actual nature and quantity of radioactive material found on the clothes. As mentioned previously, this information can be pertinent in determining the person's exposure.

The decontamination facility must also include provisions for the washing of the contaminated person's body. This station may involve the use of a portable shower unit designed to operate from fire plug water, or it may have a self-contained water supply. Portable basins and plastic water jugs may be used for washing requirements not calling for the complete bathing of the individual. With locally contaminated areas on an individual, particularly when the contaminants are highly radioactive, bathing the entire body may only result in the spread of the contaminants to the remainder of the body. Hence, careful localized washing techniques should be used wherever possible. During washing and showering, efforts should be directed toward collection of the wash liquid, not only to prevent spread of contamination, but also to provide samples. Samples, like the retained clothing, would be available for future study in determining the extent of the exposure.

The technique for decontamination of the person involves simple washing of the individual or area of his body, preferably only with water and commercially available detergents and soaps. Highly alkaline soaps, abrasives, organic solvents, or cleaners that tend to increase the rate of absorption of the contaminant into the body must be avoided. Special emphasis should be given to cleaning the fingernails, toenails, nostrils, scalp, ears, and body folds. After the person has been well washed and the contamination removed to the maximum extent of the method employed, he must be resurveyed with portable radiation monitoring instruments. Additional wipes and smears may need to be taken with disposable tissues, cotton-tipped swabs, or filter paper, evaluated, and again retained for possible re-examination or analysis. Repeated baths or washes should be made until no further reduction of the contamination is possible. The decontamination facility must be prepared to supply fresh clothing or other suitable temporary body coverings for decontaminated individuals.

The setting up of the decontamination facility at the site of a radiological accident will be a difficult task, and every possible consideration should be given to the preparation of emergency portable equipment. The consequences of the use of such facilities under adverse climatic conditions must be weighed against the harm done by delay in decontamination if the decision is made to seek a more sheltered or more comfortable area. The spread of contamination from the locale of the emergency to the decontamination station must also be considered in making such a decision.

If the decontamination facility is set up within a particular building, an evaluation of the ventilation in the room to be used must be made prior to conducting decontamination operations. This is necessary not only from the standpoint of spread of contamination to other parts of the building, but because there is the possibility of creating airborne contamination within the room itself as the result of the operations. The hazard to decontamination personnel is obvious.

Contamination of the air supply must be considered also if the facility is to be located near the site of a potential radiological accident. Preplanning and design of filter systems can reduce this potential hazard to acceptable levels.

The operation of the facility by the decontamination team personnel must be such as to minimize the contamination of these men. Proper protective clothing, gloves, caps, shoe covers, and protective respiratory devices must be provided, and controlled to prevent contamination of the facility operators. The men will probably have to undergo some decontamination themselves.

In summary, the decontamination of uninjured personnel is a complex problem. Its nature and extent will vary in the many diverse situations in which such operations must be conducted. It is sufficient to note that to select the best of the many possible actions available will require competent evaluation of each circumstance through experience coupled with technical know-how and good judgment.

The purpose of this discussion has not been to provide a stepwise operating procedure for carrying out the techniques of decontamination of uninjured personnel, but to point out the critical requirements for preplanning of such operations and for the preparation of and assembly of equipment and portable facilities, and to emphasize the need for thoroughly and completely trained decontamination personnel. In addition, it is to highlight the necessity for coordination and communication between the special teams responsible for the decontamination effort and the teams responsible for the total situation encountered at a radiological incident or accident.

This discussion has refrained from any attempt to define radiological guides, limits, or measurements which identify the need for decontamination of uninjured personnel or limits below which persons can be declared free from contamination. Such guides are published and available. In particular, reference is made to the *National Bureau of Standards Handbook 48,* entitled "Control and Removal of Radioactive Contamination in Laboratories." This discussion is aimed at re-emphasizing that a given set of rules cannot cover all situations. Such rules can, and should, only be applied by persons with good judgment and a competent grasp of the technical aspects of the radiation problem itself, as well as of the methods and techniques of monitoring and decontamination.

DISCUSSION

Chairman D. M. Gardiner (U.S. Atomic Energy Commission, Chicago) : I have a question. In the decontamination of personnel, one has to consider climatic conditions, and I ask you, what would one do in zero degree weather if you wished to have people take their clothes off?

Mr. R. H. Burr: I think such circumstances would warrant finding a more comfortable facility.

At our plant we process uranium. We live with personnel contamination all the time. This has entailed the building of shower rooms and change facilities because we use these facilities every day regardless of the weather.

MEDICAL MANAGEMENT OF CONTAMINATED PERSONNEL WITH WOUNDS OR PERSONS INTERNALLY CONTAMINATED

GEORGE L. VOELZ*

Health and Safety Division
Idaho Operations Office
U.S. Atomic Energy Commission
Idaho Falls, Idaho

THE ADVENT of extensive use of radioisotopes in industry, medicine and research brought immediate recognition of a major problem in the successful utilization of atomic energy, namely, the health hazards associated with exposure to ionizing radiation and radioactive materials. Adequate notice of the potential hazards of internal radio-emitters was given in the middle 1920's when numerous cases of severe anemias and destructive lesions of the mouth and jaw were discovered in radium dial painters. Scientific committees, such as the International Committee on Radiological Protection (ICRP) in 1928 and the U.S. Advisory Committee on X-Ray and Radium Protection (now named the National Committee on Radiation Protection and Measurements [NCRP]) in 1929, were established soon thereafter for the purpose of studying available data in order to recommend permissible radiation exposures to personnel. The radium dial painters, and patients receiving radium salts medically during these early years are the principal persons known to have suffered pathological effects due to accidental internal deposition of radioisotopes. This restricted incidence is certainly a tribute to the conscientious work of the scientists who promoted health protection during the early developmental period of atomic energy. The inhalation of high concentrations of radioactive materials (radon or radon daughters) in unventilated mines became a suspected cause of increased lung cancer in miners during the 1920's and 1930's. This is the other major group in which

*The opinions expressed in this paper are those of the author and are not intended to reflect the official position of the U.S. Atomic Energy Commission.

the pathological changes caused by exposure to internal emitters are now unquestioned.

Our greatest body of experience to date on the effects of internal emitters has been derived from the early radium exposures. Studies on the long-term effects of radium continue to take advantage of the rare opportunity presented by the rather large number of persons exposed to long-lived internal emitters (40). Our present maximum permissible limit for bone-seeking isotopes is based on a comparable energy release as delivered by a maximum permissible body burden of 0.1 μg radium-226 plus daughters (27). It is of interest that, in some 300 individuals bearing a significant body burden of radium-226, no bone tumors have been found where the total *terminal* body burden was below 0.4 μg radium-226 from exposures thirty years or more ago (40). The initial dose in a therapeutic series of intravenous radium injections was often 100-300 μg or more (22). It is suspected that the initial amount of radium in the body is a much more important factor in the carcinogenic process than the terminal body content.

Attention should be drawn to the fact that internal emitters have not produced pathological effects as a result of acute, accidental exposures. The radium dial painter exposures occurred over a period of months or years while therapeutic radium injections were received over a period of weeks. The lung exposures of the miners occurred during long occupational exposures with an average latent period of seventeen years before development of lung cancers (7). In situations where there has been uncontrolled exposure to mixed fission products following nuclear detonations, as in the case of the Marshall Islanders (8) and the Japanese fishermen (17), the exposure from the internal emitters was low and insignificant compared with the dose received from the external radiation. Workers in the atomic energy industries to date have not experienced acute accidental exposures to internal emitters which have resulted in radiation injury similar to the direct external radiation exposures which produce the dramatic acute radiation syndrome. The concern regarding internal emitters is related more to the continuing internal radiation dose which may produce late pathological effects. This concern does, in fact, assume the urgency of an emergency because of the need for rapid evaluation and early administration of therapy if any reduction in the body burden is to be effected.

A brief review of a few fundamental factors which influence the radiation dose from internal emitters may serve as an introduction upon which to base a discussion of the medical management of acute internal radioisotope exposures. Any radioactive chemical entering the body, whether through the skin, pulmonary or gastrointestinal tract, becomes an internal emitter. It continues to irradiate the tissues until it is either excreted by some physiological process, principally through the urine or feces, or until it becomes inactive through radioactive decay.

The excretion rate and amount in the urine and feces have been the principal method of estimating the burden of internal emitters. It has been customary to state the excretion rate by either exponential or power function equations in order to express its relationship to the concentration of the radioisotope present in the body and the time elapsed since exposure. Unfortunately, excretion radioanalysis admits of considerable error due to individual as well as day-to-day variations. A larger number of samples improves the accuracy of the estimate of body burden, but an average estimate may still be off by a factor of three or four (49). Obviously, the use of one or two samples following an exposure will have still larger possibilities of error; it can serve only to guide an educated guess. Despite these handicaps, excretion data serve as our principal measurement for body burdens of alpha-particle and pure beta-ray emitters.

The determination of body burdens of gamma-emitting isotopes has received a very significant advance through the use of whole-body counting techniques (24). These determinations are reasonably precise and extremely sensitive, as indicated by their ability to determine the normal body content of natural radioisotopes, such as potassium-40.

Each isotope has a specific physical radioactive half life (physical half life) as well as an independent metabolic rate of disappearance from the body (biological half life). The effective half life of the isotope in the body is derived by combining these two disappearance rates as follows:

$$\text{Effective Half life } (T_{eff}) = \frac{\text{Physical half life} \times \text{Biological half life}}{\text{Physical half life} + \text{Biological half life}}.$$

The internal emitter will be metabolized according to its chemical properties. Some radioisotopes, such as sodium-24, will become generalized throughout the body like its stable isotope. Other radioisotopes, such as iodine-131, will be concentrated in a particular organ, which thereby becomes the so-called "critical organ." Examples of the critical organs for a few elements are listed in Table III-1. These and others are found in the reports of the NCRP (27) and the ICRP (25).

TABLE III-1
CLASSIFICATION OF SOME RADIOELEMENTS (SOLUBLE FORMS) BY CRITICAL ORGANS

Bone	*Thyroid*	*Gastrointestinal Tract (GI)*	*Total Body (Generalized)*
Phosphorus	Iodine	Ruthenium	Carbon
Calcium	Astatine	Silver	Sodium
Strontium		Rare Earths	Zinc
Radium		Cobalt	Cesium
Plutonium			

Obviously, the internal dose will also be determined by the physical properties of the radiations emitted by the particular radioisotope. The alpha-particle sources become particularly important internal emitters due to the intense ionization occurring within the short range of the particles. Likewise, the shorter-range internally emitted beta particles produce relatively more intense ionization than do gamma rays with their lower specific ionization values. It has been demonstrated biologically that alpha-particle emitters are more toxic internally than the same microcurie quantity of beta emitters (10). These various physical characteristics of the radiations are an important factor in the calculation of the maximum permissible body burdens recommended by the NCRP and ICRP.

It is apparent that the evaluation of the hazards associated with the internal deposition of radioisotopes is very complex. The principal factors which must be considered will be the amount of isotope absorbed and retained in the body, the character and effective energy of the radiations, the effective half-life, and the distribution within the body with particular reference to critical organs.

Returning to the practical problems facing the physician in the medical management of internal radiocontamination cases, we may divide the problem conveniently into four phases: planning and preparation, case evaluation, decision for treatment, and treatment management.

I. Planning and Preparation

The degree of success in treating internal emitter exposures will have some direct relationship to the thoroughness of planning and preparation. We should expect to spend far more time on preparation than on actual treatment. A few specific items in regard to the internal emitter exposure problem can be briefly mentioned.

A. ***Instruments for Contaminated Wounds.*** The instruments which one should have available to evaluate potential wound contamination should include two Geiger-Mueller type survey meters. A high-range survey meter, reading in roentgens per hour, should also be available. A ⅜-inch end-window detector probe, which may be attached to a portable rate meter, has proved to be very practical in our dispensary for localizing radioactive particles on the skin and wound margins (Figure III-1). The sensitivity of this instrument is more than adequate for decontamination of beta-gamma ray emitters. In the case of one employee, after decontamination of multiple abrasions and embedded foreign bodies containing mixed fission products on the forehead and cheeks, it was still possible to localize four or five separate areas of radioactivity on the face of the patient with this small end-window probe. It was determined by whole-body counting techniques that the total residual activity consisted of only 0.02 μc cesium-137 and 0.01 μc cesium-134.

Special scintillation needle probes have been custom fabricated at some atomic energy installations (13). They are designed for accurate localization within the deeper recesses of a wound. Their application in practice has been very limited.

Alpha-particle survey instruments should be available for use by the medical department if the potential for alpha-particle emitter contamination exists. Perhaps it is unnecessary to mention that alpha-particle instruments are useful only for surface contamination free of shielding films of water or blood. A negative alpha-particle reading over a wound is only presumptive evidence that no alpha-particle emitter contamination is present.

The very toxic alpha-particle emitter, plutonium-239, can be successfully detected in surface wounds by measuring the emission of its low-energy gamma rays (38, 39). This is possible only with a special monitoring instrument consisting of a thin, thallium-activated

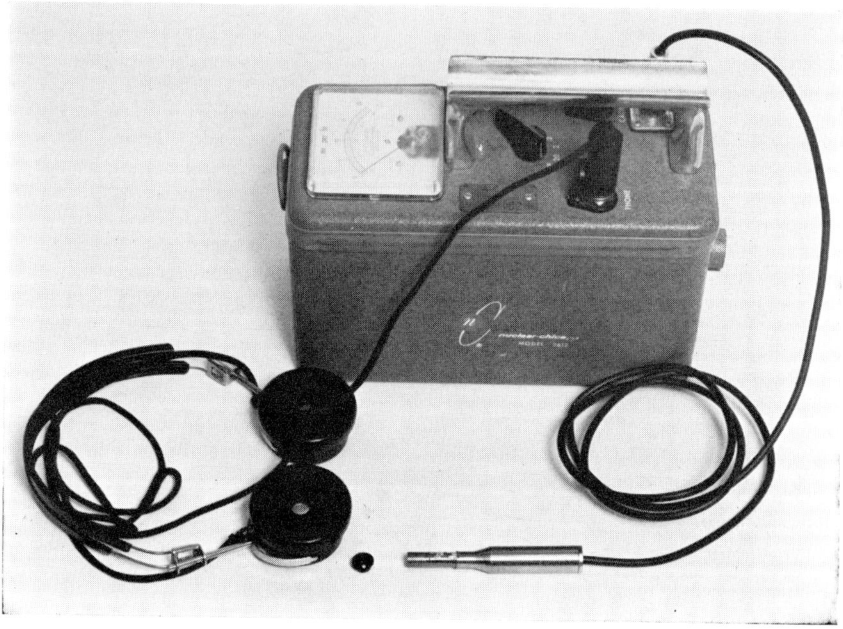

FIGURE III-1. A small, ⅜″ end window probe connected to a portable rate meter serves as a useful tool for localizing small beta-gamma ray emitting particles on skin surfaces or in wounds.

sodium iodide crystal, collimators, and a spectrometer. It is invaluable for quantitatively detecting and estimating plutonium-239 deposits within about 1 cm. of the skin surface.

B. ***Analysis for Internal Radiocontamination.*** An important part of the preparation for emergencies involving internal emitters is the study and evaluation of methods available for estimating body burden, including bioassay of excreta as well as whole-body counting techniques (28). Although the physician will probably not be responsible for making these determinations, he must be familiar with the limitations and potential margins of error in these procedures for realistic interpretation. There is no difference between this and recognition of the inaccuracies and statistical deviations present in standard clinical laboratory procedures. In addition, the physician must recognize the biological variations which may be present, particularly in early excretion data following acute exposures.

The analyses of the pure beta-ray and alpha-particle radioisotopes usually require chemical separations and preparations. The length of time required for analytical results may be considerable; for example, at least four hours for strontium-90 and sixteen hours or more for plutonium-239. These time delays preclude recourse to this type of information for use in evaluating the need for the early, first-aid type treatment. In these cases, the immediate treatment decision may have to be based on estimates of field contamination and the physical factors of the accidents. This is practical only for treatment procedures which involve no risk to the patient. Other forms of therapy must wait for more quantitative data.

A fairly recent development is the effective use of external counting techniques for beta-ray emitters, such as strontium-90. Recent data (47) suggest that 8 nanocuries of strontium-90—yttrium-90 represent the minimum amount detectable by external counting methods. An estimated standard error of 20-25 nc due to variations in the disintegration rates of potassium-40 and cesium-137 represents about 1/80 of the maximum permissible body burden for strontium-90 (2 μc) recommended by ICRP. This holds hope for more convenient, sensitive detection systems for other radionuclides emitting beta rays of equal or greater energy than those of yttrium-90.

The gamma ray emitters can be identified and counted very quickly with direct whole-body counting techniques (24). A rough localization of the activity, such as determining whether the deposit is in the respiratory tree or in the gastrointestinal tract, may be obtained by placing the scintillation crystal over these areas and comparing the relative levels of activity. The presence of high-level skin contamination may interfere; however, skin decontamination usually should be adequate to allow reasonable estimates to be made. It should be emphasized that shielded whole-body counters are designed specifically for maximum sensitivity. In accidental, brief exposure such sensitivity is not required; in fact, it may be a disadvantage if the upper limit of the counter range is reached.

The effectiveness of screening-type whole-body counters which are of simple design and without heavy shielding should not be overlooked. Figure III-2 shows such a counter recently assembled by the Health and Safety Instrument Branch, Idaho Operations Office. It is a 3 x 3 inch, thallium-activated, sodium iodide crystal surrounded by a

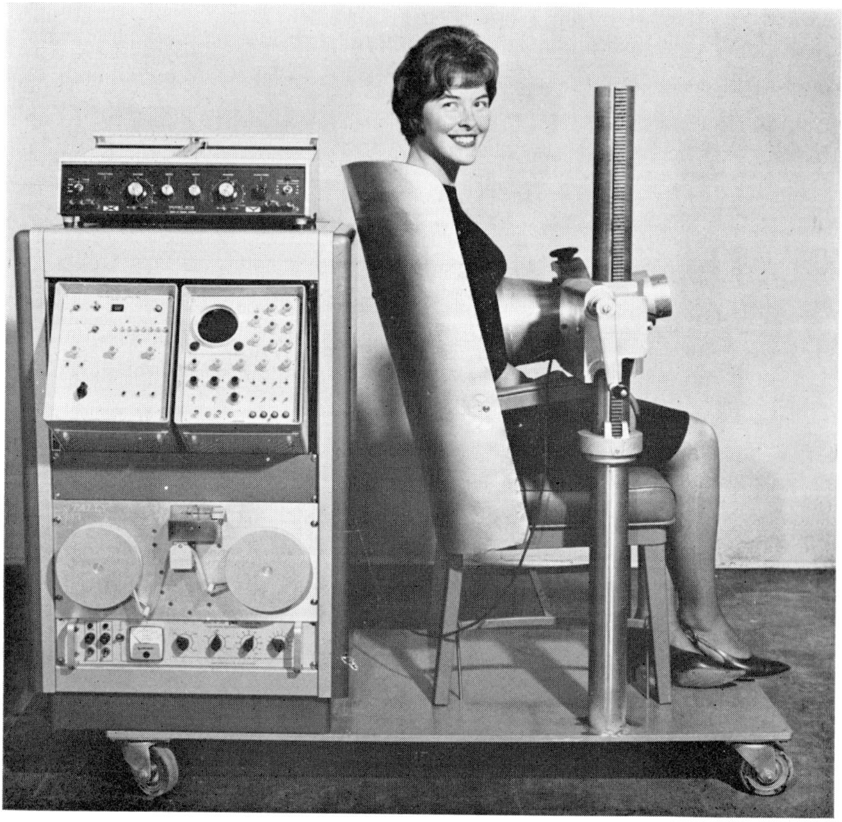

FIGURE III-2. This "light weight" gamma ray counter utilizes a lead shield around the crystal and a lead "shadow" shield behind the subject.

¾-inch lead shield. Counting devices ranging from a simple count rate meter or scaler to a multi-channel spectrometer can be used with the detector. The latter offers greater sensitivity and isotope identification, although it is more costly. The difference in sensitivity of the unshielded apparatus compared to an "iron room" type counter is in the range of a factor of 10. The instrument as presently designed is capable of detecting 0.01 μc of cesium-137 dispersed in a volume approximating the shape of the human torso. It has been estimated (47) for similar-type apparatus that 110 of 240 radioisotopes listed by the ICRP have gamma-ray emissions suitable for detection at maximum permissible body burden levels.

C. ***Special Preparations.*** The need for preliminary preparations at the hospitals for management of radionuclide contamination has been adequately discussed elsewhere (see pages 122 to 130) as well as in other publications (41).

For treatment of internal emitters, one should insure the availability of the particular drugs one may anticipate using. Unless pre-ordered, the most common and best known chelating drug, Ca-EDTA (calcium ethylene-diamine-tetraacetic acid), may even be a missing item in the average hospital pharmacy. The newer chelating drugs, like Na_3-Ca-DTPA (trisodium calcium diethylene-triamine-pentaacetic acid), are still handled as experimental drugs.

II. Case Evaluation

The complexity of evaluating a particular exposure due to an internal emitter was previously mentioned. If the particular isotope is identified, the physician should obtain information as to its physical and chemical properties as well as its known metabolic or physiologic fate. In addition, the physician will want to determine the following factors:

1) The mode of exposure.
2) Internal dose or body burden estimate.
3) Clinical evaluation of the patient.

Internal radioisotope exposures will ordinarily not create clinical symptoms in a patient. There will usually be a history of a few essential details describing an accidental exposure of an individual to a single radioisotope or possible mixture of radioisotopes. The initial steps of evaluating the situation by a general survey of the individual with either beta-gamma ray or alpha particle survey instruments, or both, will probably have been carried out near the scene of the accident. In this case, a summary of the rough preliminary readings should be obtained from the individual who made the survey. If the patient has not been surveyed, this should take precedent unless an obvious life-saving first-aid procedure is necessary. If at all possible, external contamination of the skin should be removed before the patient is transported to the medical unit.

As soon as the magnitude of external contamination has been evaluated, the next step is to obtain a clear understanding of the historical events of the accident from the patient as well as from firsthand witnesses. This will usually reveal sufficient information so that a clinical impression can be established regarding the mode of exposure and its relative seriousness. Thus the probability of an ingestion exposure versus an inhalation exposure may be apparent if an accurate description of the accident and the type of radioactive material is available. These determinations, coupled with field survey readings, may be sufficiently impressive to consider proceeding with a no-risk, first-aid treatment without delay. In a few instances, treatment has been carried out within ten to thirty minutes of an accidental exposure (48). First-aid treatment of this type must be set up at the work site in order to be applied so rapidly.

Further evaluation of the case will now proceed with positive identification of the radioisotope involved and determination of the body burden by direct counting techniques and bioassay of excreta. The significance of these determinations should be reviewed in the light of the particular mode of exposure and the particular radionuclide. A limited discussion of this type of evaluation is presented for illustrative purposes.

A. ***Intact Skin Absorption.*** The most frequent radiocontamination problem in industry, research, and medical laboratory involves the intact skin. The "insoluble"* isotopes will not penetrate the intact skin barrier, and will not become internal emitters via the skin. However, the soluble isotopes, such as iodine-131, will pass the skin barrier. Radiostrontium chloride in a neutral solution has been found to penetrate intact, shaved rat skin (21). Soluble salts of uranium, as distinguished from insoluble uranium forms, have been shown to penetrate the skin (35). Tritium water has been found to exchange through the skin at about the same rate as it would cross the pulmonary membranes. Therefore, it is necessary to wear plastic suits if tritium-contaminated atmospheres are likely to contact the skin.

Acidic and alkaline solutions will increase the permeability of the skin since the integrity of the skin barrier is altered. Plutonium salts ordinarily will not pass through the skin; however, in two instances, internal exposures occurred when plutonium in acid solutions contacted the skin (19, 20).

*Throughout this paper reference is made to solubility or insolubility in water, not in body fluids, lungs, etc.

B. ***Wound Contaminations.*** Any physical break in the continuity of the skin accompanied by radiocontamination may introduce radionuclides to the dermis, subcutaneous and underlying tissues. This problem of contaminated wounds has not presented any particularly serious difficulties up to now as far as beta-gamma ray emitters are concerned. The ability to detect beta and gamma-ray activity in wounds simplifies the problem of identification and localization.

The presence of alpha-particle emitters in wounds has been a problem of genuine concern to industry. Their detection and localization present considerable difficulty, although the detection of associated low-energy gamma-ray emissions has improved the ability to detect and localize superficial plutonium deposits. The prospect of long-lived irradiation of subcutaneous tissues as well as significant systemic absorption of plutonium demands removal of all detectable amounts of this contaminant from wounds, if possible. It has been demonstrated (5) in swine that 70 per cent of an intradermal dose of plutonium-239 nitrate remains at the site after eight days, but less than 2 per cent is left at 565 days. The importance of prompt detection and treatment of such deposits is apparent.

In addition to absorption and translocation, there is the problem of continuous irradiation of local dermis or subcutaneous tissue which may produce neoplasms. Lushbaugh (23) reported the excision of a skin nodule containing 0.078 μg of plutonium which had been deposited there for fifty-one months. Precancerous epidermal changes were noted secondary to a rather fantastically high radiation dose which was estimated to be 75 million rads at the surface of the deposition.

C. ***Inhalation Exposures.*** Inhalation of radioactive particulates or aerosols has been the most common and important source of internal deposition in atomic energy installations. The deposition and absorption of radionuclides via the lung is an extremely complex subject which is only partially understood. A good summary of our current knowledge has been published by the National Academy of Sciences (16).

The deposition of material in the respiratory tract depends on the physical properties of the aerosol as well as on the anatomical and physiological characteristics of the recipient. Impaction is a principal factor determining the deposition in the upper respiratory tract where the moderately large particles (5-30 micron) remain. Sedimentation of the smaller particles (0.5-5 micron) is particularly important in the lower respiratory tract where the air velocity is low. Diffusion or Brownian motion is important in the deposition of the smallest particles (less than 0.1 micron). Thus, as the particle size increases beyond a few microns, deposition increases in the upper and decreases in the lower respiratory tract. The greatest fraction deposited in the respiratory tract consists of particles of about 2-micron size and goes through a mininum in the 0.2 to 0.5 micron range. Fast, shallow breathing results in less deposition than slow, deep breathing if other factors are equal.

The retention, clearance, and translocation of inhaled particles are primarily determined by physiological processes. Particles are removed from the respiratory tract in at least four ways: ciliary action, transfer of soluble material across the alveolar membrane, phagocytosis, and physical transport of particulates through lung tissue. An initial lung clearance rate due apparently to ciliary action has a half life ranging from hours to several days (3), while a slower process from deeper portions of the respiratory tract has a half life from several days to months, depending on the particular material (18). These clearance rates are an important factor in determining the radiation dose to the pulmonary tissues. A major portion of the material is transported up the respiratory tract and removed via the gastrointestinal tract. The ICRP standard lung model (25) uses a conservative basis for dose calculations assuming that, with "soluble" particles, 25 per cent are exhaled, 50 per cent are deposited in the upper respiratory tract and transported to the gastrointestinal tract, and 25 per cent are taken up in the body via the lower respiratory tract. The model assumes that "insoluble" compounds follow the same pattern, except that only 12.5 per cent is taken up in body fluids via the lower respiratory tract, with a 120-day half life. An additional 12.5 per cent is assumed to be transported up the respiratory tract and swallowed within twenty-four hours.

Phagocytosis of particulates is an important clearance mechanism. Some phagocytes are transported up the respiratory tract, but a significant fraction also enters the lymphatic vessels and is transported to the pulmonary lymph nodes. For this reason, the critical organ for "insoluble" particles, especially alpha-particle emitters, may be the pulmonary lymph nodes.

The fate of the inhaled radioisotope is partially determined by its solubility in body fluids. Although this is largely dependent upon its chemical composition, it is also determined by the physical properties of the particle, such as size, shape, and surface area. In the case of induced radionuclides, as may occur around reactors or particle accelerators, the particles may consist of a matrix of various materials with physicochemical properties different from those usually associated with the radionuclide in question.

Experience at the National Reactor Testing Station has indicated the frequency with which airborne radionuclides inhaled around nuclear reactors act primarily as insoluble material (42). The exposures occurred as a result of low-level (deposition usually of less than 1 μc, with a maximum of 2.6 μc) inhalation incurred by reactor operating personnel. Studies of these gamma-ray emitting isotopes included whole-body counting as well as radioanalysis of urine and feces. Of twenty different radionuclides encountered, only iodine-131, -132 and -133, cesium-137 and -134, mercury-197 and -203, and molybdenum-technetium-99 were excreted in urine sufficiently for detection by routine gross gamma-ray counting of spot urine samples. Zinc-65, silver-110, ruthenium-103 and -106, and cobalt-60 were eliminated primarily via the feces, although they were infrequently detected in the urine using large (1500 ml) volume samples and sensitive counting techniques. The radionuclides eliminated entirely via the gastrointestinal tract and never detected by urinalysis consisted of chromium-51, zirconium-niobium-95, antimony-22, manganese-54, cerium-141 and -144, and barium-lanthanum-140. The radionuclides eliminated via the gastrointestinal tract were observed to have biological half lives varying from sixty-five to 295 days, which presumably represent the clearance rates of these particular insoluble particles from the lower respiratory tract. These studies point out the inadequacy of radiological urinalysis for detecting the inhalation or ingestion of radionuclides which may be in an insoluble physicochemical form.

The case study following inhalation of radionuclides should include whole-body counts, radiological urinalysis, and fecal analysis. The follow-up should be continued for a sufficient period of time so that the biological half life can be determined as accurately as possible. There is need for this type of data on most of the internal emitters. Whole-body counting has proved to be particularly useful for measuring internal contamination from gamma-ray emitters and for determining their biological half life.

D. ***Ingestion Exposures.*** Ingestion is not often encountered as the primary type of exposure in occupational accidents, with the glaring exception of the radium dial painters. This mode of exposure is more important in chronic exposures through food or water supplies, such as might occur in heavy fallout situations either from nuclear weapon detonations or possibly in the environs of a major plant disaster. All inhalation exposures have a significant ingestion component, as was previously noted.

Factors influencing gastrointestinal-tract exposure include the chemical form ingested, the characteristics of the radiation emitted, the residence time in the tract, the mixing and combination of the radionuclide and gut contents, the state of being fasted or fed prior to ingestion, and the ability of the isotope to cross the intestinal epithelium. Hayes and Carlton (14) have studied the individual variations of dose from beta-particle emitters to the lower large intestine. The dose may differ by as much as a factor of five from that of the ICRP standard man assumptions in 6 per cent of the population, and a factor of three times the standard in 15 per cent. In experiments on dogs and goats, the dose from non-absorbable, beta-ray emitting yttrium-90 compounds was about twelve times greater with constipation than with diarrhea (29). The importance of understanding these factors better can be appreciated when one realizes that the gastrointestinal tract is the critical body organ for more than 50 per cent of the 230-plus radionuclides listed in the NCRP and ICRP publications. More specifically, the critical organ is generally the lower segment of the large intestine, where the gut contents remain for about 75 per cent of the time required for passage through the entire gastrointestinal tract.

The solubility of the radionuclide compound in question within the gastrointestinal-tract environment determines the systemic absorption which will occur. A highly soluble compound, such as iodine, will be absorbed entirely into the systemic circulation. Other radionuclides are partially absorbed, such as ruthenium-106 which has an absorption of about 3 per cent; some are, for all practical purposes, passed without absorption, e.g., plutonium with a 0.003 per cent absorption fraction. The rare-earth nuclides are not absorbed through the gastrointestinal tract. Spencer and Rosoff (46) indicate that 90 to 100 per cent of an oral dose of "soluble" $Y^{91}Cl_3$, $La^{140}Cl_3$ and $Sc^{46}Cl_3$ is recovered in the feces of man, with none detected in the urine and plasma.

E. ***Biological Samples.*** A most important detail from a practical medical viewpoint is the advisability of collecting all biological excreta, including urine, feces, and vomitus. A 10 ml blood sample taken during the earliest hours following the accident should be saved for radioanalysis. No particular preservatives are required for these samples.

It has been customary to take nose swipes for radioanalysis, but experience indicates that they are of no practical value for correlation with the magnitude of exposure. A positive result simply indicates the likelihood of an exposure. Solutions used to irrigate the nose and mouth should be saved, however.

III. Decision for Treatment

It is self-evident, in view of the complexities of evaluating internal radiocontaminants, that the decision as to whether or not to treat a patient will be complex. Unfortunately, the time of greatest efficiency of all treatment procedures is the earliest possible hour after exposure. This obviously is also the period of least information upon which to base medical decisions.

The information in this early time period will perhaps consist of some scanty information on the accident, probable identification of the major radioisotope by history, and no clinical symptoms or signs. The probable complete absence of clinical features places the physician at a great disadvantage in trying to determine the need for immediate treatment. An immediate survey for radiocontamination is the first physical measurement which may indicate the magnitude of the accident. The physician will not wait for a long period of study for better dose calculations before making his immediate decisions. These decisions will be based on rough estimates, past experiences, clinical appraisal, and medical judgment. Admittedly these are vague, indeterminant quantities which defy definition, but which are not unknown in other medical decisions. There may be past experience with the isotope in question which suggests that safe preventive and treatment procedures should be instituted immediately. The risk of any therapy must be balanced with the available information defining the risk of a particular exposure.

Within a relatively short period, it should be possible to perform direct counting procedures for gamma-ray emitters, and to obtain urine and blood samples for radioanalysis. On the basis of these, it should be possible to arrive at a rough estimate of the radiation dose. This initial appraisal may be adequate for considering further treatment methods, such as the administration of chelating agents.

The estimate of the prospective radiation dose to the critical organ will determine the necessary action. The physician must evaluate the "probable" risk to the patient. This is really a statistical probability as to whether biological effects may occur within the patient's lifetime. This evaluation cannot be made entirely by correlation with the listed maximum permissible body burdens (MPBB) listed by the NCRP (27) or the ICRP (25). The MPBB is determined by the radiation dose delivered to the critical organ if this body burden is maintained for the working lifetime (50 years) of the individual. It is intended for evaluation of prolonged exposures rather than isolated, brief exposures. The effective half-life of the isotope becomes a vital factor in a single, brief exposure. A long-lived internal emitter, such as plutonium-239 ($T_{eff} = 64,000$ days) or strontium-90 ($T_{eff} = 6400$ days), will deliver a significant lifetime burden. A short-lived isotope, such as iodine-131 ($T_{eff} = 7.6$ days) has such a short exposure time to the critical organ that the risk involved must be evaluated in terms of the total integrated radiation dose to the critical organ rather than reference to the MPBB.

IV. Treatment of Internal Radionuclides

A. ***Wound Decontamination.*** The first consideration of the physician should be his concern for the patient's general welfare. The application of immediate emergency procedures to control hemorrhage, to restore respiratory and circulatory function, and to alleviate pain is obviously a first order of business even if it requires significant radiation exposures to recovery and medical personnel. It is advisable to establish in advance the upper exposure limit to which recovery and medical personnel may be exposed for lifesaving purposes. An exposure limit of 100 rad has been considered acceptable in some emergency plans (15). The NCRP recommendations (26) include a once-in-a-lifetime, 25-rad emergency exposure which need not be applied to the individual's occupational exposures.

It will be only in exceptional cases that such high beta-gamma ray contamination levels face the physician. Relatively minor wounds with a surrounding area of low or moderate radiation readings are much more probable. The decontamination of the wound will, almost without exception, begin with immediate rinsing of the wound under running tap water in such a manner that the water flows away from the wound. The application of an arterial tourniquet is generally considered a desirable procedure to reduce absorption into the systemic circulation. This procedure is of greater importance for the more soluble isotopes. The contaminated areas of surrounding skin are cleaned by use of the conventional decontamination agents used on intact skin—detergents and water, a nylon bristle brush for scrubbing, abrasive soaps, titanium dioxide powder, kitchen cleansers, special abrasive pastes, potassium permanganate followed by sodium bisulphite for stain removal, dilute acids or complexing agents like citric acid or sodium ethylene-diamine-tetraacetic acid (EDTA). Care must be exercised to prevent these solutions from entering the wound. Radiological monitoring determines the extent of these decontamination activities.

The wound is treated in such a manner that conventional surgical aseptic conditions are maintained. The decontamination procedures on the surrounding skin may serve also as a presurgical scrub. Necrotic tissue is surgically removed. If the wound still contains significant contamination, a block resection of the entire wound will generally be the procedure of choice. Since these wounds are most frequently on the hands, the surgeon may not be able to excise them completely without creating functional disability. It would be an unusual contamination which would require consideration of such sacrifice.

The excision of contaminated wounds has been practiced most frequently when plutonium-239 was the contaminant. The very low permissible body burden and long effective half life require complete removal of this isotope so that excision of the area has been the only practical solution. The beta-gamma ray isotopes do not present the same degree of hazard and, to my knowledge, excision has not been required in any such cases.

B. ***First Aid for Ingestion Procedures.*** During the initial concern for the identification and dose estimation of the radionuclide involved in an accident, the physician should not overlook the prospect of using such simple expedients as irrigation of the nose, mouth and pharynx, the removal of gastric contents, and the use of purgatives. These are practical procedures that can be employed immediately without risk to the patient and without special equipment. Any reduction of the residence time of the radionuclides in the gastrointestinal tract will reduce the dose proportionately, as well as decrease the time during which absorption can take place. The time for effective action is very short. Bruce (4) indicates that absorption of the soluble portion of ruthenium, for example, is essentially complete within one hour, even though a high percentage of the insoluble portion may be retained on the wall of the small intestine for several hours. Any "soluble" radioisotopes will probably have been absorbed completely within only thirty to sixty minutes. The induction of vomiting by mechanical stimulation, or the use of a stomach tube and pump is the most immediate and effective means available to remove the stomach contents. The use of an emetic, such as zinc sulfate, ½ gm in a glass of warm water, or by injection of 1/12 gr apomorphine may also be considered.

Certain simple chemical antidotes have been suggested and used as first aid administrations to reduce the absorption of certain ingested radioisotopes. Volf (48) has shown that oral barium sulphate administration can be effective following acute radiostrontium ingestion. He further suggests that oral barium sulphate can probably be used effectively for the accidental ingestion of radioisotopes of calcium, barium, and radium. Magnesium sulphate has also been suggested as a desirable oral agent for these isotopes, because of its well-known laxative action as well as the chemical action of the sulphate radical.

Calcium phosphate and phytates may be of value following ingestion of radiostrontium. Experimentation on their relative effectiveness and possible combinations needs to be carried further.

The use of a laxative, such as 10 gm of magnesium sulfate in 100 ml of water, will reduce the exposure in the lower segment of the large bowel. This should be considered with unusually large exposures to insoluble materials traversing the gastrointestinal tract.

C. ***Immediate Procedures for Inhalation Cases.*** Inhaled radionuclides which are soluble in body fluids will be absorbed by the lung very rapidly. No first-aid procedures are effective here except such preventive action as holding one's breath if in a presumed high concentration of these radionuclides. Additional therapy must be directed toward increasing excretion from the system or reducing the uptake in the critical organ.

It seems possible that one may be able to stimulate the lung clearance mechanisms where relatively "insoluble" radioisotopes are involved. Unfortunately, this is a treatment area which has only recently begun to receive attention experimentally. Guidelines for human therapy are, therefore, almost nonexistent. Initial studies have shown that the simultaneous administration of relatively large quantities of inert dust (carbon black) with small amounts of insoluble uranium dust increases the lung clearance rates (18). The use of negative ion therapy has also been reported to speed up the ciliary beat and mucus flow. Bair *et al.* (2) were unable to confirm any effectiveness of either inert carbon black aerosols or negative ions in promoting lung clearance of radioactive particles in rats. During a follow-up study (42) of an inhalation exposure to silver-110, a marked decrease in body (lung) burden was noted during a period of coughing associated with a "cold." This may suggest that lung clearance processes can be accelerated.

Bair *et al.* (2) tested the effectiveness of using an aerosol of a chelating drug, diethylene-triamine-pentaacetic acid (DTPA), to treat animals exposed to $Ce^{144}O_2$ dust, a relatively insoluble compound. This treatment reduced the lung burden of cerium-144 -praseodymium-144 to less than 10 per cent of the amount in untreated animals. The same treatment was only slightly effective against $Pu^{239}O_2$ and plutonium nitrate aerosols. A surface-active agent, Pluronics F 68, was found to increase urinary and fecal excretion of inhaled plutonium in dogs and rats more effectively than did chelating aerosols of DTPA and TTHA (triethylene-tetraamine-hexaacetic acid).

These early experimental data do not lead us to any practical medical regimens. Certainly, if any aerosol-type therapy is to be effective, it will require administration as soon as possible after exposure. Part of the medical preparation for treating inhalation exposures to radionuclides may be the consideration of various forms of aerosol therapy which can be given without undue risk to the patient.

D. ***Systemic Treatment for Several Radioisotopes.*** Up to now, the discussion has dealt with therapy which may limit the extent of absorption of radionuclides at the point of initial contact with the body. The treatment of systemic burdens of radionuclides is of limited effectiveness, but may offer an additional significant dose reduction for some radioisotopes.

To date, systemic treatments which have proved to be of some value include the administration of: 1) stable compounds which are competitive with the radionuclide for uptake in the critical organ; 2) drugs which stimulate some physiological function to reduce residence time of the radionuclide in the system, and 3) chelating agents which form soluble metal complexes to increase the excretion rate of certain radioisotopes. The application of these methods to a few specific radioisotopes is briefly reviewed in order to illustrate the principal techniques available.

1. RADIOIODINE. An example of dose reduction in the critical organ by the use of a competitive stable isotope is the administration of a stable iodide to reduce the uptake of radioiodine in the thyroid gland. The increase in available iodides reduces the percentage of radioiodine uptake in the thyroid gland even if administered several hours after the exposure. Adams and Bonnell (1) estimate that 100 mgm of stable iodide should reduce the thyroid radiation dose by a factor of 5 to 10. Their recommended adult oral dose is 100 mgm of potassium iodide immediately after the exposure, and repeated in four hours. Daily doses should be administered as long as significant radioiodine activity

is still evident. A major advantage of the use of a stable iodide is its negligible toxicity and wide range of safety. It may be considered even for administration to the general public if a release of radioiodine encompasses a large geographic area such as might occur following a major reactor accident.

The administration of antithyroid drugs, such as propylthiouracil, methimazole, or carbimazole will reduce the radiation dose in the thyroid by reducing its retention of radioiodine and preventing organic binding of iodine to form the specific thyroid hormones. Potassium thiocyanate and potassium chlorate also effectively inhibit the thyroid's absorption of inorganic iodide from the plasma. Although the antithyroid drugs are potential bone-marrow depressants, they may be preferred to stable iodides in cases where high exposures have occurred, and where the patient is under medical supervision.

2. Tritium. Tritium, a radioactive hydrogen isotope, diffuses readily throughout the body water. The increased turnover of body water will flush out the tritium at an increased rate. Pinson (37) was able to decrease a ten-day biological half life to approximately 2.4 days by forcing 12.8 liters of water per day in one individual. The treatment of this radionuclide therefore holds the tantalizing prospect of forcing beer as a therapeutic agent, radiologically as well as psychologically speaking. The use of diuretic drugs also holds prospects for dose reduction.

3. Radiostrontium. The removal of absorbed radiostrontium has not been highly successful to date; however, it appears to be possible to influence the normal physiological functions involved to some extent. It has been found that there is a qualitative relationship between the urinary excretion of calcium and radiostrontium. Efforts to enhance the excretion of calcium in urine have effectively increased the excretion of radiostrontium. This effectiveness decreases as the period between the exposure and the treatment is increased; however, some effect is still noted several weeks after exposure. Spencer (44) found intravenous calcium gluconate (470 mgm Ca^{++}) and oral ammonium chloride (9 grams daily) to be effective when given immediately, and even two weeks after exposure. In one of three patients, the body burden was less than 10 per cent of the administered dose after twelve days, compared to the control value of 44 per cent. Intra-

venously administered stable strontium was more effective than equivalent amounts of calcium.

The chelating agent BAETA (bis 2-aminoethyl ether tetraacetic acid), given intravenously, will approximately double the excretion rate of radiostrontium during the first twenty-four hours (45); it is also effective in the late phase, i.e., two weeks after exposure (44). Zirconium citrate and sodium calcium citrate have also been reported to be effective against radiostrontium. Zirconium does have toxic properties—immediate nausea and vomiting with subsequent development of vertigo—and is not a very desirable agent for use in man. Tests with other chelating agents, EDTA and DTPA, have been unsuccessful for use with radiostrontium.

4. TRANSURANIC ELEMENTS (PLUTONIUM, AMERICIUM, CALIFORNIUM AND NEPTUNIUM). There has been more experience with the treatment for the removal of plutonium in man than with treatment for other radioisotopes. The principal treatment has consisted of the use of intravenous administration of chelating agents, originally EDTA, and more recently, DTPA (30-33). The administration of DTPA will increase the urinary excretion of plutonium by a factor of 50 to 100. If treatment starts immediately after exposure and the source of exposure to plutonium can be eliminated, such as with wound excision, it appears that about 65 per cent of the body burden will be eliminated over a period of six months or so (34). A reasonable treatment schedule in man is to give 1 to 1½ gms of Na_3-Ca-DTPA intravenously in 250 cc of isotonic saline or 5 per cent glucose on each of three days, beginning as soon after the exposure as the decision for treatment can be made. After a week or two, a similar administration of DTPA would be repeated. The need for additional periodic therapy will depend on the estimate of the body burden, analysis of the excretion rate, and the effect of DTPA administration on the excretion rate. Apparently, small amounts of DTPA remain in the body and will continue to enhance the excretion rate for a period of three months or more. There have not been serious side effects noted in man at these dose levels. Reversible kidney tubular damage has been described by Foreman (11) after the use of both EDTA and DTPA. Routine clinical urinalyses should be carried out during chelation therapy for early recognition of this potential effect. Renal disease may constitute a contraindication for the use of these drugs.

Americium has been successfully treated with EDTA in one human case (12). It was estimated that the body burden after treatment was less than 10 per cent of what it would have been without treatment. DTPA produced a five- to seven-fold increase in urinary excretion of both americium-241 and californium-252 in mice, using a dose schedule comparable to those recommended for human therapy (36).

DTPA has also been effective in reducing the retention of californium-252 and neptunium-237 in rats (43).

5. RADIORUTHENIUM. Ruthenium is chelated efficiently by 1:2-Bis-[2-di (carboxymethyl) amenoethylthio] ethane (BATE) (6). There is a minimal practical value in the use of this chelating agent due to the extremely slow dissociation of ruthenium-protein complexes. Therefore, the extent of mobilization of ruthenium is very small if the chelate is administered after ruthenium has been absorbed.

6. RARE EARTHS (CERIUM, YTTRIUM, LANTHANUM, SCANDIUM). Both DTPA and TTHA (triethylene-tetraamine-hexaacetic acid) are effective therapeutic agents for use in the removal of internally deposited cerium-144 (6). It was found to be effective even if treatment was started after a delay of a few days. In rats, the skeleton and kidney burden was reduced to 60 to 80 per cent of control animals, while the liver burden was reduced to about 20 to 50 per cent of the controls (6). These results were obtained with DTPA treatment beginning three to thirty-one days after injection of $Ce^{144}Cl_3$. The effectiveness of treatment was greatest with the shortest interval before therapy.

Yttrium-90, lanthanum-140 and scandium-46 can be effectively removed in man by using the chelating agents EDTA and DTPA (46). DTPA is more effective and appears to be the preferable agent for therapy of rare-earth internal depositions. DTPA therapy increased scandium-46 excretion rates in one individual to twenty to fifty times the pretreatment values (46). The increased excretion rates continued for several days after treatment.

REFERENCES

1. Adams, C. A., and Bonnell, J. A.: Administration of Stable Iodide as a Means of Reducing Thyroid Irradiation Resulting from Inhalation of Radioactive Iodine. *Health Physics,* 7:127-149, 1962.

2. Bair, W. J., Tombropoulos, E. G., and Park, J. F.: Distribution and Removal of Transuranic Elements and Cerium Deposited by the Inhalation Route, in *Diagnosis and Treatment of Radioactive Poisoning.* Proc. of WHO and IAEA Scientific Meeting, Oct. 15-18, 1962, Int. Atomic Energy Agency, Vienna, pp. 319-338, 1963.
3. Brieger, H., and LaBelle, C. W.: The Fate of Inhaled Particulates in the Early Postexposure Period. *Arch. Ind. Health, 19*:510-515, 1959.
4. Bruce, R. S.: Some Factors Influencing the Absorption, Retention, and Elimination of Ruthenium, in *Diagnosis and Treatment of Radioactive Poisoning.* Proc. of WHO and IAEA Scientific Meeting, Oct. 15-18, 1962, Int. Atomic Energy Agency, Vienna, pp. 207-224, 1963.
5. Cable, J. W., Horstman, V. G., Clarke, W. J., and Bustad, L. K.: Effects of Intradermal Injections of Plutonium in Swine. *Health Physics, 8*:629-634, 1962.
6. Catsch, A., and Seidl, D.: Rare Earths and Ruthenium: Metabolism and Removal from the Mammalian Body, in *Diagnosis and Treatment of Radioactive Poisoning.* Proc. of WHO and IAEA Scientific Meeting, Oct. 15-18, 1962, Int. Atomic Energy Agency, Vienna, pp. 191-205, 1963.
7. Claus, W. D., ed.: *Radiation Biology and Medicine.* Addison-Wesley Publishing Co., Inc., Reading, Mass., p. 350, 1958.
8. Cohn, S. H.: Metabolism of Fission Products in Man: Marshallese Experience, in *Diagnosis and Treatment of Radioactive Poisoning.* Proc. of WHO and IAEA Scientific Meeting, Oct. 15-18, 1962, Int. Atomic Energy Agency, Vienna, pp. 235-251, 1963.
9. *Diagnosis and Treatment of Radioactive Poisoning.* Proc. of WHO and IAEA Scientific Meeting, Oct. 15-18, 1962, Int. Atomic Energy Agency, Vienna, 1963.
10. Finkel, M. P.: Late Effects of Internally Deposited Radioisotopes in Laboratory Animals. *Radiation Res.,* Suppl. No. 1, pp. 265-279, 1959.
11. Foreman, H.: Discussion on Renal Damage from Chelating Agents, in *Diagnosis and Treatment of Radioactive Poisoning.* Proc. of WHO and IAEA Scientific Meeting, Oct. 15-18, 1962, Int. Atomic Energy Agency, Vienna, pp. 379-380, 1963.
12. Foreman, H.: Medical Management of Radioactively Contaminated Wounds, in *Diagnosis and Treatment of Radioactive Poisoning.* Proc. of WHO and IAEA Scientific Meeting, Oct. 15-18, 1962, Int. Atomic Energy Agency, Vienna, pp. 387-411, 1963.
13. Hathaway, E. A., and Finkel, A. J.: Medical Care of Wounds Contaminated with Radioactive Materials. *J.A.M.A., 161*:121-126, 1956.
14. Hayes, R. L., and Carlton, J. E.: Radiation Dose to the Human Intestinal Tract from Internal Emitters. Report ORINS 42, Oak Ridge Institute of Nuclear Studies, 1962.
15. Horan, J. R., and Gammill, W. P.: The Health Physics Aspects of the SL-1 Accident. *Health Physics, 9*:177-186, 1963.

16. Kornberg, H. A., Chairman, Subcommittee on Inhalation Hazards: *Effects of Inhaled Radioactive Particles.* Publication 848, National Academy of Sciences—National Research Council, Washington, D.C., 1961.

17. Kumatori, T., and Miyoshi, K.: Clinical Studies on Persons Injured by Radioactive Materials, in *Diagnosis and Treatment of Radioactive Poisoning.* Proc. of WHO and IAEA Scientific Meeting, Oct. 15-18, 1962, Int. Atomic Energy Agency, Vienna, pp. 253-272, 1963.

18. LaBelle, C. W., and Brieger, H. G.: Synergistic Effects of Aerosols; II. Effects on Rate of Clearance from the Lung. *Arch. Ind. Health, 20*:100-105, 1959.

19. Lister, B. A. J., Morgan, A., and Sherwood, R. J.: Excretion of Plutonium Following Accidental Skin Contamination. *Health Physics, 9*:803-815, 1963.

20. Lister, B. A. J., Morgan, A., and Sherwood, R. J.: *Excretion of Plutonium Following Accidental Skin Contamination.* U. K. Atomic Energy Research Establishment, AERE Report 4064, 1962.

21. Loeffler, R. K., and Thomas, V.: *A Quantitative Study of Percutaneous Absorption*—Absorption of Radiostrontium Chloride in Minute Quantities Through the Intact and Mechanically Damaged Rat Skin. U.S. Naval Radiological Defense Laboratory, Report AD-225 (B), 1950.

22. Lucas, H. F., Jr., Rowland, R. E., Miller, C. E., Holtzman, R. B., Hasterlik, R. J., and Finkel, A. J.: An Unusual Case of Radium Toxicity. *Am. J. Roentgenol., Radium Therapy and Nucl. Med., 90*:1042-1051, 1963.

23. Lushbaugh, C. C., and Langham, J.: A Dermal Lesion From Implanted Plutonium. *Arch. Dermatology, 86*:461-464, 1962.

24. Meneely, G. R., ed.: *Radioactivity in Man.* Charles C Thomas, Publisher, Springfield, 1961.

25. Morgan, K. Z., Chairman, ICRP Committee II: *Permissible Dose for Internal Radiation.* ICRP Publication 2, Pergamon Press, London, 1959.

26. NBS Handbook 59, *Permissible Dose from External Sources of Ionizing Radiation.* Recommendations of the NCRP, U.S. Government Printing Office, Washington, D.C., 1954.

27. NBS Handbook 69, *Maximum Permissible Body Burdens and Maximum Permissible Concentrations of Radionuclides in Air and in Water for Occupational Exposure.* Recommendations of the NCRP, U.S. Government Printing Office, Washington, D.C., 1959.

28. NBS Handbook 80, *A Manual of Radioactivity Procedures.* NCRP Report No. 28, U.S. Government Printing Office, Washington, D.C., 1961.

29. Nold, M. M., Hayes, R. L., and Comar, C. L.: Internal Radiation Dose Measurements in Live Experimental Animals, II. *Health Physics, 4*:86-100, 1960.

30. Norwood, W. D.: Early Diagnosis and Treatment of Individuals Who Have Excessive Depositions of Radioisotopes. *J. Occupational Med., 4*:373-382, 1962.

31. Norwood, W. D.: Long-Term Administration of DTPA for Plutonium Elimination. *J. Occupational Med.*, *4*:130-132, 1962.

32. Norwood, W. D.: Removal of Plutonium and Other Transuranic Elements from Man, in *Diagnosis and Treatment of Radioactive Poisoning.* Proc. of WHO and IAEA Scientific Meeting, Oct. 15-18, 1962, Int. Atomic Energy Agency, Vienna, 1963, pp. 307-318.

33. Norwood, W. D.: Therapeutic Removal of Plutonium in Humans. *Health Physics, 8*:747-750, 1962.

34. Norwood, W. D.: Personal Communication.

35. Orcutt, J. A.: *Pharmacology and Toxicology of Uranium Compounds.* National Nuclear Energy Series, McGraw-Hill Book Company, New York, p. 377, 1949.

36. Parker, H. G., Low-Beer, A. de G., and Isaac, E. L.: Comparison of Retention and Organ Distribution of Am^{241} and Cf^{252} in Mice: The Effect of *in vivo* DTPA Chelation. *Health Physics, 8*:679-684, 1962.

37. Pinson, E. A.: *The Body Absorption, Distribution and Excretion of Tritium in Man and Animals.* Los Alamos Scientific Laboratory, Report LA-1218, 1951.

38. Putzier, E. A., Mann, J. R., and Johnson, V. P.: Use of a Gamma Ray Spectrometer for Investigation of Plutonium Contaminated Wounds. *Am. Ind. Hyg. Assoc. Quarterly, 19*:384-385, 1958.

39. Roesch, W. C., and Baum, J. W.: Detection of Plutonium in Wounds. *Proc. 2nd U.N. Int. Conf. PUAE,* Geneva, *23*:142-143, 1958.

40. Rowland, R. E.: Local Distribution and Retention of Radium in Man, in *Diagnosis and Treatment of Radioactive Poisoning.* Proc. of WHO and IAEA Scientific Meeting, Oct. 15-18, 1962, Int. Atomic Energy Agency, Vienna, pp. 57-68, 1963.

41. Saenger, E. L., ed.: *Medical Aspects of Radiation Accidents.* U.S. Government Printing Office, Washington, D.C., 1963.

42. Sill, C. W., and Anderson, J. I.: Comparison of Excretion Analysis with Whole-Body Counting for Assessment of Internal Radioactive Contaminants, To be published.

43. Smith, V. H.: *Biology Operations Monthly Report.* Hanford Atomic Products Operation, HW-73905 D, Page D3, May 1962.

44. Spencer, H.: Removal of Radiostrontium from Man, in *Diagnosis and Treatment of Radioactive Poisoning.* Proc. of WHO and IAEA Scientific Meeting, Oct. 15-18, 1962, Int. Atomic Energy Agency, Vienna, pp. 145-155, 1963.

45. Spencer, H., Feldstein, A., and Samochson, J.: Effect of the Chelating Agent Bis 2-Aminoethyl Ether Tetraacetate (BAETA) on Radiostrontium Excretion in Man. *J. Lab. Clin. Med., 59*:445-455, 1962.

46. Spencer, H., and Rosoff, B.: Metabolism and Removal of Rare Earths in Man, in *Diagnosis and Treatment of Radioactive Poisoning.* Proc. of WHO and IAEA Scientific Meeting, Oct. 15-18, 1962, Int. Atomic Energy Agency, Vienna, pp. 171-189, 1963.

47. Vennart, J.: External Counting, in *Diagnosis and Treatment of Radioactive Poisoning*. Proc. of WHO and IAEA Scientific Meeting, Oct. 15-18, 1962, Int. Atomic Energy Agency, Vienna, pp. 3-22, 1963.
48. Volf, V.: Treatment of Radiostrontium Uptake in Man, in *Diagnosis and Treatment of Radioactive Poisoning*. Proc. of WHO and IAEA Scientific Meeting, Oct. 15-18, 1962, Int. Atomic Energy Agency, Vienna, pp. 131-144, 1963.
49. Williams, K.: *Bioassay of Excreta and Body Burden of Radioactive Materials*. U. K. Atomic Energy Research Establishment, Report AERE-R3288, 1960.

MAXIMUM PERMISSIBLE LEVELS FOR INTERNAL CONTAMINATION

GEORGE V. LeROY

Department of Medicine
The University of Chicago
Chicago, Illinois

THE TITLE assigned to me has an important implication that I wish to point out. The implication is that there should be special guidelines for emergency exposure from internally deposited radioactive material comparable to the "permissible emergency dose" of 25 rads of external whole-body gamma radiation. I cannot accept this, and can think of no sufficient reason to use any other guidelines than those outlined in NCRP-NBS *Handbook 69* (1).

During the actual accident that creates the radiation emergency, some or all of those involved may acquire—by inhalation, ingestion or absorption—an internal deposit of radionuclides. This deposit, however, is not subject to control—and hence the term "permissible" cannot be applied to it—any more than one can speak of "permissible traumatic injuries." When, and if, one knows the dose received from internally deposited material, I believe this dose should not be excluded from the exposure record of the victim. In most accidents which I can imagine, I would expect the external dose to be much larger than the dose equivalent due to internally deposited material. Nevertheless, I do not think it should be ignored in record-keeping.

In the controlled phase of an emergency, we all agree that it will be necessary to authorize selected personnel to perform tasks which involve exposure to external radiation in excess of the maximum permissible occupational dose, but in an amount that should not exceed 25 rads. Since this emergency exposure can be controlled, it is my opinion that the officials in charge should require that all emergency personnel use whatever protective devices are necessary to prevent, or drastically limit, any inhalation, ingestion, or absorption of radioactive material. (Of course, in case of accidental failure of the protective equipment, the above conditions will not have been met.) Administrative supervision of emergency exposure to external radiation will be difficult enough in most cases, and it seems to me the height of folly to complicate matters by attempting to keep a running estimate of emergency internal exposure in relation to some permissible level.

The position which I have taken does not mean that I attach no significance to internal exposure. The fact is that I believe the most strenuous efforts are justified to quantitate the body burden of radionuclides acquired during an emergency. This is not the same, however, as saying that we should establish a "permissible emergency burden, or dose." As I said before, I think that very strong efforts should be made by all concerned to minimize or prevent internal deposition of radioactive material *after* the uncontrolled phase of the emergency.

The standard operating procedures for a peacetime radiation emergency should include clear and simple provisions for obtaining information that will permit evaluation of the nature and the extent of radioactive material deposited internally. I have examined several emergency plans and am not entirely satisfied with any of them.

At this point, I want to digress somewhat to comment on the handling of injured people whose skin and clothing are contaminated, and who may or may not already have internally deposited material as a result of inhalation, absorption, etc. According to most plans, those who escape or are removed from the site of a radiation accident go first to a health physics station. Some plans stipulate that health physics personnel, after monitoring a casualty and removing contaminated clothing, will carry out certain decontamination measures, even to the extent of washing out wounds, abrasions, etc. Depending on the circumstances, this may be contrary to good medical practice. If a physician or qualified industrial nurse is available, he should inspect each casualty with the health physicist, and the doctor or nurse should decide whether or not decontamination should take precedence over first aid or over definitive emergency treatment. When a doctor or industrial nurse is not available, health physics personnel should limit their medical activities to the removal of contaminated clothing, the washing of superficial abrasions, and the washing out of the eyes.

In the case of those with serious injuries, e.g., lacerations, fractures, stretcher cases, concussions, etc., another procedure should be mandatory: Lacerations should be covered with sterile compress bandages, emergency splints should be applied to fractures, the degree of contamination should be noted on the emergency medical tag; and the victim, wrapped in a protective covering, should be transferred at once to a hospital. I am very deeply concerned that time spent in monitoring and decontamination of uninjured skin, hair, etc., will increase the risk of shock and other well-known complications of traumatic wounds. I am also concerned about possible deleterious effects of over-enthusiastic cleansing of lacerations and other large wounds by the use of strong detergents and other decontamination agents.

Obviously, a thoroughly contaminated injured person creates problems for the staff of the average hospital where definitive care can be given. Nevertheless, good cooperation with health physics personnel should minimize most difficulties and restrict the spread of radioactive contamination. Doctors, nurses and attendants can wear protective clothing, and their contamination can be controlled without interfering with proper medical care. The point I wish to make is that, with few exceptions, a serious wound takes precedence over radioactive contamination.

I shall now consider procedures to evaluate the nature and the amount of internally deposited radioactive material. The most important thing at the outset is to collect all urine passed by each person from the time he escapes—or is removed—from the site of the accident. Depending on the circumstances, radioassay of the first urine voided may be of great value, or it may contribute little to an estimate of the accidental burden of radioactive material. The length of time during which total collection of urine should continue will vary; however, a decision should be made on this point as soon as possible, because even so simple a thing as collecting all urine involves some difficulties. The same rule applies to emergency personnel who enter the contaminated area for any reason: all the urine which they pass should be collected.

Unfortunately, we have very little precise information about the relationship between rate of urinary excretion and body burden for most radionuclides. Thus, the results of radioassay of urine may allow only order-of-magnitude estimates. Identification of nuclides excreted should not present a serious problem in a well-equipped laboratory. After the initial level of activity in urine has been estimated, suitable aliquots should be frozen for later detailed study. On the basis of my experience, I suggest that it is most convenient to collect individual voidings in pint-size plastic bottles. In each case, the hour and date of voiding, and the subject's name should be recorded.

I fail to see any benefit from examination of feces, and recommend that this procedure be deleted from emergency manuals. The same is true for sputum, saliva, nasal secretions, and what not. If a person has been caught in a radioactive cloud, all these samples will contain activity. These samples are rarely used except as a general indication of exposure. If the radioactivity in the cloud is known, one can calculate with reasonable accuracy the dose received by the individual exposed to it. The cloud is an external rather than an internal source of radiation. There, too, I fail to see any benefit in taking sputum, saliva, and nasal secretion wipes because I know of no way to relate the radioactivity of the cloud to the activity of these samples. In most peacetime accidents, there will be enough to do without devoting time and effort to collection of data which cannot be used in any meaningful fashion.

At some time after an accident, the wounds of the victims will be dressed, skin and hair will be decontaminated, and there should be reports on the radioassay of the urine of the first few days. At this time, one or two courses may be followed. If radioiodine was among the nuclides accidentally released, serial monitoring of the thyroid gland should be started. The results ought to give a fair estimate of the extent of internal contamination since the thyroid acts as a trap for iodine. If the thyroid contains no iodine-131 after an accident involving a reactor or a critical assembly, the probability is very small that there is any significant deposit of other nuclides. If the thyroid contains any iodine-131, it will be worthwhile to arrange for whole-body counting at some institution which has a gamma-ray spectrometer. We have had some experience with ingested insoluble particulate radioactive material, and can state with confidence that, in most people, more than 99 per cent will be excreted during the first six days after ingestion of a single dose. It is probably not wise to put a person in a whole-body counter until wipe tests of skin demonstrate that decontamination is complete.

In order to facilitate whole-body counting, I would not hesitate to prescribe laxatives to hasten the elimination of radioactive material from the intestinal tract.

Once the skin is clean, and after, say, six days, the results of a whole-body count should provide a reliable measurement of the amount and kind of radionuclides retained. Serial counts allow one to follow excretion at times when radioassay of urine and feces would be difficult. Knowing the nuclides retained, and their effective half-life, the calculation of dose equivalent from internally deposited material is straightforward.

To the extent that it is possible, I would recommend this procedure not only for those involved in the actual accident, but also for the personnel of the emergency crews, clean-up people, etc. As I mentioned earlier, everyone who enters the contaminated area during the controlled phase of the emergency should be required to collect all the urine passed from the time he is assigned to this duty. Prompt assay of such urine at the end of each shift will allow the health physicist in charge to detect evidence of absorption of activity due to faulty use or failure of respirators and other protective devices. If I were the man in charge, I would make the collection of urine a condition of employment equal in importance to the use of safeguards and the wearing of dosimeters. No urine—no job!

In most emergencies which I can imagine, the procedure that I have outlined should allow the health physicist to evaluate the extent of the body burden of radionuclides acquired during the emergency. He should then be able to calculate a dose equivalent in rem resulting from the activity deposited internally. I have not suggested that any added internal deposit should be considered permissible—and I recommend the the dose equivalent resulting from the emergency should be included in the worker's exposure record. I am sure that, in serious accidents, the combined internal and external doses received by some people will substantially exceed not only the regular occupational median lethal dose (MLD), but also the National Committee on Radiation Protection and Measurements (NCRP) emergency dose.

REFERENCE

1. NBS Handbook 69, *Maximum Permissible Body Burdens and Maximum Permissible Concentrations of Radionuclides in Air and in Water for Occupational Exposure*. Recommendations of the NCRP, U.S. Government Printing Office, Washington, D.C., 1959.

HOSPITAL PREPAREDNESS FOR HANDLING CONTAMINATED PERSONS REQUIRING MEDICAL CARE

ROBERT S. LANDAUER, SR.

Cook County Hospital
Chicago, Illinois

HOSPITAL PREPAREDNESS for handling contaminated persons must be simple and uninvolved if it is to have any chance of success. It must not be loaded down with minutiæ, and it cannot be expected to cover all possible situations. It is a plan for an emergency, and the "comforts of home" and the niceties of normal existence cannot be included.

Preparedness involves far more than a mere stock-piling of instruments and materials, important as this is. A list of materials and instruments is given as an appendix to this paper (Appendix III-1).

Proper preparedness must include a thorough understanding, by both the administrative and the medical staffs, of the problems involved. The answers to most of these problems must be determined on a local basis. They depend on the philosophy of the staffs, the physical facilities of the hospital, and the magnitude of the available intern, resident physician, nursing, and lay personnel groups. The problems to be solved fall into the categories of what is to be done, who will do it, where it will be done, and what tools will be required. This last is comparatively easily answered; the others, not so easily.

The principal purpose of this paper is to acquaint the staffs with the problems involved, so that they can discuss and resolve them in advance of an emergency. These discussions should be arranged in consultation with some expert in radiological safety, be he the radiologist, the isotopologist, or an outside guest.

The need for authoritative help in the planning stage is illustrated by a story recently told to me: A large part of the staff of a big hospital was amazed to learn that accident victims of a cobalt-60 gamma-ray overexposure were not themselves radioactive, and did not require decontamination.

It should be stated here that this discussion is not to be construed as a plan for dealing with a military holocaust; such, I think, would be impossible to handle for most civilian hospitals. Plans may be made, however, for the sorting and reception of a hundred or so victims, 30 per cent of whom may be contaminated.

One of the most important measures in preparedness planning is for the hospital to know upon whom to call for help when an emergency arises. The hospital superintendent or administrator, upon receiving word that patients involved in a radiation accident will be arriving shortly, should get in touch immediately with one or more of the following:

1) The Department of Radiology of the nearest large hospital.
2) Any known qualified health physicist or health physics organization in the area.
3) The U.S. Public Health Service.
4) The health physics section of any nearby Atomic Energy Commission facility.
5) The local Health Department.
6) The State Department of Health.
7) The local Medical Society.
8) The local office of Civil Defense.

Those of the above who respond affirmatively should be asked to come themselves, or to send representatives to the hospital as quickly as possible, and to bring with them any simple survey meters which they may have, and which are in current operating condition.

When the injured arrive at the admitting station, they will have to be surveyed for radioactivity before being admitted into the hospital for triage. This is not in order to determine whether or not they are contaminated, for any instrument reading above background would indicate contamination, but to ascertain whether the degree of contamination is sufficient to warrant decontamination procedures before instituting medical treatment. There seems to be no unanimity of opinion on this subject. I have been told, "If the survey meter registers anything over background, the victim must not be allowed to enter the hospital." I have also been told, "If the victim has a gash in his femoral artery and is bleeding to death, he should be taken into the hospital regardless of contamination." These are extreme views. I think that the answer to this will depend much on the degree of injury, the degree of emergency, and the philosophy of the medical staff of the individual hospital.

There are some available figures (see Table III-2) for maximum permissible skin and clothing contamination which do not require any decontamination (1). These figures contain a large factor of safety and are designed for use under normal operating conditions. By how much may these numbers be exceeded in a disaster-type emergency? It is clear that no single figure can be used, but it is also obvious that to attempt to have a different number for each different condition would be completely unrealistic. This is the kind of minutia which must be avoided. A rational approach might be that, if the subject does not require immediate medical attention, an off-scale reading on the lowest scale (0.5 mR/hr) of a civil defense type beta-gamma ray survey meter would be the criterion for requiring decontamination before admittance to the hospital. Under emergency medical conditions, 100 mrad per hour might be used. This is a number sometimes accepted for admittance to an air raid shelter before decontamination is required.

A subcategory of the measuring problem is that of instrumentation. It is no doubt true that the vast majority of accidents will only involve exposure to beta- and gamma-ray emitting isotopes. However, there is always the possibility of alpha-particle emitter contamination which, if undetected and not removed, can be very serious, especially to the victim himself. There seems to be a prevalent idea that those at the site of an accident will not only know immediately exactly what happened, but will communicate this information to all the hospitals, so that the person with the survey meter at admittance will be alerted to look for "a man in a green suit who may have received alpha-particle emitter contamination." I think that this is completely unrealistic and that, in most instances, information regarding specific types of contamination will not be available at the sorting centers. A center must be in a position to measure at least the three common types of radiation which may be encountered. I would hate to be in the position of having filled a room with "radiologically clean" patients, to find later that some of them were thoroughly contaminated with an alpha-particle emitting nuclide. I think that the staffs should consider the additional cost of alpha-particle surveying well worthwhile.

It may be noted that I have included alpha-particle survey meters at both sorting and decontamination areas. A quite moderately priced alpha-, beta-, gamma-ray Geiger-Mueller survey probe which can be readily connected to a rate meter of the civil defense type is commercially available. Its use would eliminate many of the drawbacks of the more sophisticated types of alpha-particle detectors.

Who is to do the sorting of contaminated and uncontaminated individuals? It must be by members of some group which is on duty at all times, every day and every night. From the above discussion, it is evident that it is desirable for medical judgment to accompany meter reading. Hence, the sorting should be done by physicians. In a large hospital, such a medical group might be the intern or resident pool from which physicians at the admitting office are drawn. One or more of this group are always at the admitting station. In the small hospital, the problem is more acute, and physicians may simply not be available for this purpose; therefore, lay meter readers will have to be employed. In this case, a simple rule such as the following must be established for the initial sorting: "If the pointer stays on the lowest scale, admit the patient. If it goes off the lowest scale, hold the patient and call for a medical opinion." This will not work under all conditions, but nothing will work under all conditions; some plan must be worked out which can be lived with.

These people will have to be trained to use simple survey meters, with special emphasis on ability to recognize the uncertainties of correct operation of such instruments. This training will of necessity be a continuing operation, being repeated with changes in personnel. I think that a one-hour lecture demonstration once a month by either the radiation safety officer or the radiologist would provide adequate training.

Who is to see to it that the instruments are in operating condition at all times, and that they are within reasonable calibration limits? This might well be a duty assigned to the chief x-ray technician or to the isotope technician, assuming, of course, that a health physicist is not on full or part-time duty. Instruments should be checked at regular intervals, and such inspections indicated on a card attached to the instrument, much as is done with fire extinguishers.

If possible, patients should be surveyed inside the vehicle in which they are delivered. Patients to be decontaminated should remain in the delivering vehicle, and be immediately transported to the entrance to the decontamination area. Large signs should be posted at admittance indicating the location of, and the route to, the decontamination area. In the event of a high background in the vehicle, patients should leave the vehicle one at a time and be surveyed in the open. Those found to require decontamination should be returned to the vehicle.

Assuming that decontamination is necessary, where will it be done and by whom? A proper program means getting the victim to the decontamination area and decontaminating him, all without further spread of radioactive material. An outlying building such as a garage would be ideal. In the absence of such a room, space in a basement might serve, provided the logistics of transporting the patients to this space are not too involved. Morgues and autopsy rooms may be considered.

The room or area provided for decontamination must have showers, or at least stalls where the patients can be hosed down with running water. It is desirable, but by no means necessary, that separate washing facilities be provided for male and female patients. Deep sinks are most convenient. They should preferably be located near the floor, to aid in the washing and scrubbing of extremities. The designated room should be stocked with the supplies listed in the Appendix (Appendix III-1).

If the room is connected with a general air conditioning system, means must be provided for a "disconnect," to prevent the dissemination of radioactive material throughout the hospital. It is important always to remember to "contain" radioactive material, not to spread it. This applies to the decontamination team personnel as well. These people should not leave the area without first ascertaining that they themselves are not contaminated. There have been several instances of physicians spreading radioactivity all over a hospital and even into their homes.

The decontamination team should be composed of at least one physician, one or two registered nurses, and several attendants or orderlies. The physician should be either the radiotherapist, a general radiologist, a physician familiar with handling radioactive isotopes, or some non-radiologically oriented physician who has been taught decontamination procedures. Regular staff nurses should be assigned by the director of nursing services, and attendants and orderlies should be assigned by their supervisors. These assignments should be made as soon as the disaster plan is formulated, and reassignments should be made as required to keep the team on a currently active basis.

Written instructions for decontamination procedures should be given to and learned by all personnel assigned to decontamination duty. These instructions should be as brief as possible, and written in simple cook book style, without theory or reasons. Actual procedures are fully described in numerous publications.

TABLE III-2

MAXIMUM PERMISSIBLE SKIN AND CLOTHING CONTAMINATION

Surface or Item	*Beta, Gamma Ray mrad/hr*	*Alpha Particle $d/m/100cm^2$*
General Body	0.06	150
Hands	0.3	150
Shoes:		
Inside	0.3	300
Outside	0.6	300
Clothing	0.25	150

A word may be said regarding permissible exposure to both sorting and decontamination personnel. Pocket dosimeters should be worn. If possible, persons should be relieved of duty when their exposure reaches five rad. In extreme circumstances, the rotation level may be set at 25 rad. In general, no deleterious effects need be anticipated from an exposure of 25 rad.

Contaminated clothing and materials should be placed in large cans. When a can has been filled, it should be removed and stored in some unoccupied area until the termination of the emergency. After this, the local or State Department of Health or the U.S. Atomic Energy Commission should be contacted and the problem of what to do with the materials turned over to them.

It should be readily apparent that most of the plan lies in the hands of the local hospital staffs. My advice to them is: KEEP THE WHOLE PLAN AS SIMPLE AS POSSIBLE, AND DO NOT ATTEMPT TO MAKE IT COVER ALL CONTINGENCIES. IF YOU DO, IT WILL MOST CERTAINLY BOG DOWN, AND YOU WILL END UP WITH NOTHING.

APPENDIX III-1

Suggested supplies and instruments for use in preparedness program. Quantities may obviously be adjusted to the expected needs of the individual hospital.

At Admitting Office or Station

2 - transistorized beta-gamma ray Geiger-Mueller survey meters (Civil Defense type, non-jamming, lowest scale 0.5 mrad/hr), with one set of spare batteries for each meter.

2 - alpha-particle survey meters, with one set of spare batteries per meter. *Note:* It is possible to obtain a thin end window Geiger-Mueller probe (not to exceed 1.4 mg/cm^2 mica) which would be capable of detecting alpha, beta, and gamma rays. This could be used as the probe of the first item, and special alpha-particle survey meters could then be omitted.

6 - pocket dosimeters (0-25 rad range).

1 - charger unit for above with spare battery.

2 - 25-gallon galvanized iron or fibre cans with tightly fitting lids.

100 - tags with strings (for identification purposes).

10 - paper suits of assorted sizes.

10 - plastic suits of assorted sizes.

4 dozen - paper shoe covers.

4 dozen - plastic shoe covers.

8 - three cell-type flashlights with two sets of spare batteries for each.

1 - roll plastic tape with the standard U.S. Atomic Energy Commission insignia and bearing words, "Radioactive Material."

At Decontamination Area

2 - transistorized beta-gamma survey meters as in Item 1 above.

2 - alpha survey meters, as in Item 2 above.

1 - ionization chamber survey meter (Cutie Pie), with one set of spare batteries.
12 - pocket dosimeters (0-25 rad range).
1 - charger unit for above with spare battery.
1 - continuous alpha-beta air monitor (with spare batteries or for 110 volt alternating current operation) (optional item).
2 dozen - plastic bags (large enough to contain a patient's clothing).
4 dozen - plastic bags of various sizes, smaller than the above.
12 - plastic suits (assorted sizes).
2 dozen - paper suits (assorted sizes).
6 pair - fireman's type knee-length rubber boots (assorted sizes).
6 - respirators.
4 dozen - surgical masks.
4 dozen - surgical caps.
4 dozen - plastic shoe covers.
4 dozen - medium weight rubber gloves.
2 dozen - heavy weight rubber gloves.
3 rolls - three inch adhesive.
3 rolls - three inch masking tape.
10 - 25-gallon steel or fibre-board drums with tightly fitting lids.
2 rolls - (large size) plastic tape with the standard U.S. Atomic Energy Commission insignia and bearing words, "Radioactive Material."
1 dozen - approximately 12″ × 12″ placards, with standard U.S. Atomic Energy Commission insignia, bearing words, "Radiation Area."
1 dozen - approximately 12″ × 12″ placards, with standard U.S. Atomic Energy Commission insignia, bearing words, "High Radiation Area."
2 rolls - (standard size) 60-pound kraft paper 36 inches wide.
2 rolls - heavy plastic sheeting 36 inches wide.
1 assortment - heavy duty remote handling tongs and forceps.
1 large assortment - gowns, shoes and other clothing for patients.
6 - one-pound cans of decontaminating agent.
1 dozen - galvanized iron pails (three gallon size).
1 assortment - housekeeping items, including, but not limited to:

paper towels, soaps, scissors, paper cups, scrub brushes, cleansing tissue.

1 - basic first aid medical kit.

Drugs as determined by prior decision of hospital staff.

REFERENCE

1. Saenger, E. L., ed.: *Medical Aspects of Radiation Accidents.* U.S. Government Printing Office, Washington, D.C., 1963.

DISCUSSION

Dr. G. V. LeRoy: I wanted to make a few comments on what Dr. Landauer said, because this relates to a topic involving a good deal of discussion time at a recent seminar at the World Health Organization in Geneva, Switzerland, on protection of the public from radiation. What I wish particularly to comment on is the hospital to which victims may be taken who are contaminated with radioactivity.

I think it is a great mistake, except in thinking about transport accidents, to assume that the victims of industrial radiation accidents will go into any public hospital. I think it is important, in developing emergency plans for nuclear energy installations, to plan for the care of any injuries that may occur. This means, in a sense, making prior arrangements with certain selected hospitals in the neighborhood which could be assisted in developing a capability for taking the responsibility for the special care needed.

To send injured, contaminated people from an accident that involved radioactive material to the nearest hospital without any knowledge of whether this hospital has either the people or the capability to work with such patients, or to hospitals that had never discussed or developed emergency plans with the operators of the plant where the accident occurred, would seem to me to be the height of folly.

One of the things brought out in the Geneva meeting was that it was clearly the responsibility of the operator of the atomic energy installation—and it might very well become in many countries, especially in Europe, one of the requirements for the licensing of reactor and other sites—to develop an emergency medical plan which involved a collaborative arrangement with a nearby medical facility.

I also think it would be misconduct, or at least malfeasance on the part of the responsible operators of an industrial nuclear energy organization, to send patients to any hospital without having them accompanied by at least one or more people who are skillful in dealing with the problems of radioactive contamination. I think the responsibility clearly is upon the operators of such installations to make sure that when, in an emergency, their people have to be taken to a hospital, they go to one that is prepared, and that they go accompanied by representatives of their own organization. Now, you can envisage, on the basis of what Dr. Landauer said, that such things are much less likely to occur. The hospital would not have to depend on finding someone with a rate meter which he thought might work. And I would urge those of you who don't have plans that involve the medical facilities in the neighborhood to begin to make such plans before you have an accident.

Dr. R. S. Landauer: This is almost Utopia, I'm afraid. There is nothing I would like better than to know that every patient that came to my hospital was going to come with complete information about what had happened. I don't think this is what is going to occur. Take a transportation accident that happens in the middle of a corn field somewhere. The nearest hospital has got to have some sort of preparation for taking care of this. It may be unlikely to happen, but still it may.

I know several radium installations not too far from here where I'm sure there has not been the slightest preplanning for what would happen if there was a spread of contamination. Those accident victims are going to be taken to the nearest hospital. I think this is what is going to happen. It is not what should be done, but I think this is what is very likely to happen.

Chairman D. M. Gardiner: As a member of the U.S. Atomic Energy Commission and therefore an eternal compromiser, I am going to say something that perhaps falls midway between what we have heard. In our operation in Chicago, we are concerned with reactors that operate in the middle of corn fields. We have one in Nebraska, a very beautiful reactor in a beautiful corn field, but it sits somewhere around thirty-five to forty miles from the nearest inhabited area. We have one on the Elk River in Minnesota, and one in Ohio. In setting up our emergency plans for those reactors, we did certainly put in Dr. LeRoy's suggestion. We contacted local medical groups and hospitals.

We came to a very peculiar realization which is perhaps based on what Dr. Landauer said, and this is that the knowledge of the treatment of radiation accidents is not something peculiar to ourselves alone, but, for some reason I can't quite understand, the medical profession has managed to keep itself educated and knows that there are such things as contaminations and problems associated with contamination control. Actually, the experience we had was that we simply had to present our problem to the hospital, and in each case the hospital approached drew up, I think, very realistic programs for treatment of injured personnel and for the control of contamination.

We have had other experiences, however, particularly with parts of the industry that are not controlled by the U.S. Atomic Energy Commission, in which accident cases involving contamination have occurred. We had some accident cases involving truck drivers, and their treatment was at a local level, the nearest hospital facility; we have the problem of going in and measuring contamination and then following it from the hospital into people's homes. I think, though, predominantly the sort of plan which Dr. LeRoy has described is the one which you will find most frequently.

Dr. T. L. Shipman (Los Alamos Scientific Laboratory, New Mexico): I would like to go back and touch on one of Dr. LeRoy's statements a bit; he implied that things worth doing are worth doing well. He was referring to diagnostic measurement procedures. I think the same thing is somewhat true of the therapeutic measures which have been talked about, written about, and widely discussed. There is a tendency to play the numbers game here a little bit, and I agree that it is a perfectly wonderful intellectual *tour de force* if you can produce a body burden from just a little above the level where you have to report to the U.S. Atomic Energy Commission to a little below that level.

In an earlier paper (p. 33), Dr. Oken pointed out that one of the symptoms of the anxiety syndrome is a desire to keep doing something. I point out that this affects the personnel who are looking after the emergency as well as it does the victims of the emergency, and there are a great many radiation accidents which are not emergencies at all. Carl Unruh in his paper (p. 13) categorized four phases of radiation accidents, and called them the occurrence, emergency, recovery and restoration phases. I think there is one other phase we ought to consider. Somewhere around the recovery phase there is one which, if we want to be nice, we will call the diagnostic phase, but otherwise we will call it the phase of confusion. This is when nobody is sure whether there was an accident or not, and if there has been, how severe it is. This is the time when people are dashing in all directions wanting to do things. This is the time when, more than at any other time, one wants trained, experienced, calm personnel, and sometimes a course of inactivity is greatly to be desired.

Dr. H. Cember (University of Cincinnati): I have a comment to make about the use of the word "soluble" applied to inhaled products. The assumption is always made that the soluble product is rapidly cleared out of the lung. We have evidence, at least in rats, and I presume the same thing would be applicable to other animals, that some of the soluble material doesn't clear out very rapidly. For example, in the case of cerous ion, it could either precipitate into a very highly insoluble hydroxide, or bind to the tissue protein in the lung. In either case, we have found radiocerium that had been deposited in the lung as Ce^{144} Cl_3 solution to be retained about as tenaciously as highly insoluble Ce^{144} F_3 particulates.

As far as translocation is concerned, even up to three years after exposure to a cerium compound in the lung, we have found bronchogenic carcinoma in the lungs of these animals, and no evidence whatsoever of having damage in the bones or skeleton. The same thing would probably be true of certain other ions also. But we have got to be very careful in generalizing this point.

Dr. G. L. Voelz: Our experience around reactors has certainly been in line with your study. Material such as zinc-65 would be thought of as a very soluble material. After exposures in certain reactor situations and under field conditions, we have noticed that, following inhalation, we can find zinc-65 by whole-body counting but do not find it in the urine. The material may be in a physical matrix completely different from what you expect. We have identified at very low levels approximately 24 different types of radionuclides in people working around reactors and most of the material has been relatively insoluble.

Mr. A. V. Zila (U.S. Atomic Energy Commission, New York): Getting back to the doctors, I have a question, and maybe Dr. LeRoy or Dr. Landauer would like to answer. Perhaps emergency planning does not give individual doctors the recognition they should have, so I was going to ask, what proportion of doctors in industrial medicine are prepared to utilize the available information to help develop emergency plans? If they are few, shouldn't these doctors be sought out? And if they are many, how much should they be consulted in formulating emergency plans?

Dr. G. V. LeRoy: Your question forces one to generalize. I think we can start off by generalizing fairly accurately by stating that the ordinary industrial physician has relatively little specific knowledge for dealing with radiation injury or for evaluating the degree of contamination with radioactive material. However, he has been trained to deal with other toxic substances whose properties may differ in detail, but are similar in a general way. So, if I had my choice in working out an emergency plan, let us say, between cooperating with a hospital staff or with an industrial physician in developing a plan for emergency radiation accidents, I would prefer to deal with the industrial physician because of his philosophy of practice.

I would guess that major installations such as the big power reactors or large processing plants are unlikely to have in their vicinity hospitals with people who already have knowledge about the care needed in radiation accidents. If they are lucky, and if their location is not unusual, they are probably within thirty to fifty miles of two or more hospitals. Nowadays, transport of injured people is not much of a problem. We can move patients in modern ambulances or by helicopter very readily. I think it would be well to select from among the available hospitals the one where you can get the best cooperation and one which is located where it is easy for consultant groups, U.S. Atomic Energy Commission emergency teams, etc., to converge rapidly if you need them.

I would not have any serious concern about the ability to train a small group of people in a hospital of a hundred or two hundred beds or more, to be able to function satisfactorily with the outside help that can be provided on short notice in almost any emergency I can visualize. However, I can imagine nothing but sheer confusion created by taking a person to the nearest hospital without its having any prior information, and asking them on an *ad hoc* basis to develop a plan for dealing with a radiation accident. Radiation injuries are sufficiently infrequent in this country so that no hospital is going to have a standard radiation injury plan unless it has had a prior arrangement with a major atomic energy industrial group to take care of their people on demand. At a hospital like ours (Billings Hospital, The University of Chicago), we are prepared to do this. We have doctors identified who are prepared to put a previously established plan into operation. I would not expect just any hospital to do the same sort of thing.

Mr. A. V. Zila: Thank you. I had in mind the people already in the medical centers such as you are attached to. The midwest seems to be well prepared for this kind of accident. In some urban centers in the east, the far west, where the contractor or people doing radiation work are sort of intermediate, and where the hospital has other problems, the person doing radiation work might have to rely on some industrial-medicine-type physician for advice. I have wondered whether these people shouldn't be looking for physicians who are able to tell them what they need in the way of emergency plans, and for physicians who can utilize this information.

Dr. G. V. LeRoy: I don't know how to answer you because there is certain information I don't have. I believe that, except for some very small operations, most plants where an accident involving more than a half dozen or a dozen people could occur, or where genuine widespread emergencies would develop unless something was done promptly, are not so remote from adequate hospitals that you would have to call on inadequately prepared medical personnel or facilities to take care of your injured people.

Dr. G. L. Voelz: On the subject of hospital preparedness, I have to agree somewhat with Dr. Landauer in that I believe all hospitals should have some recognition of the nature of the problem of dealing with radiocontamination. Perhaps they don't need to be prepared for some of the major emergencies you might envision in an atomic energy plant, but they ought to know the basic principles. I believe they are willing to learn if we have people to go out and teach them.

Recently, we had a one-day seminar in Idaho Falls, which is in the far west, for hospital administrators, x-ray technicians, and most particularly for emergency room nurses. The people who attended came from unlikely hospitals such as the Blackfoot Hospital, Twin Falls, and others in southern Idaho. We had 80 people attend the conference, including many non-technical administrative people to whom we pointed out some of the problems. We concluded that there is a very serious need for radiation accident information among this type of hospital personnel. I thought that it had been widely disseminated by literature, but there were few people among this type of hospital personnel who knew that a radiation emergency plan existed. For example, if they had been faced with a transportation accident involving radioactive substances with a truck or with an airplane crash, of those eighty people only four would have known that the U.S. Atomic Energy Commission has emergency plans and that the hospitals could get help from them.

Mr. T. Fields: The American College of Radiology has recently sent to every hospital in the country a radiation disaster kit. I would venture to say that, within the next two or three years, every hospital in the country with an x-ray department that is accredited will know how to handle contaminated patients. I believe much of this discussion won't be necessary after the next two or three years, when we hope that there will be responsible people in all hospitals who will have been informed how to handle radiation accident patients.

Dr. H. Cember: Reference was made earlier to physicians trained in industrial medicine, in relation to the development of a plan for emergency radiation accidents. I want to comment on the supply of such physicians, who might make use of the various instructions and additional pieces of information handed down by the U.S. Atomic Energy Commission and others knowledgeable in radiation and radiation effects. I don't know what fraction of the total number of industrial physicians completed the postgraduate one-year training course in industrial medicine. There are about eight or ten schools around the country which have such a program, and I believe that every one of these requires a course in health physics for the doctors. This course is either one semester or a year in length. I know that this is certainly required at the University of Pittsburgh; it is also required now at the University of Cincinnati and, I believe, at all of the other institutions as well. Therefore, industrial physicians who have completed one of these training programs have more than a minimum amount of the knowledge which would be needed in order to utilize this information.

Chapter IV

RESTORATION MEASURES — BUILDINGS AND EQUIPMENT

DECONTAMINATION METHODS, EQUIPMENT AND MATERIALS

LEE GEMMELL*
Health Physics Division
Brookhaven National Laboratory
Upton, New York

In case of an accident or emergency involving radiation in a hospital, a research institution or an industrial complex, prompt definitive action must be taken to protect the workers from exposure to radiation and to confine the spread of radioactive contamination to as small an area as possible. After these safety precautions have been taken, the restoration of the buildings and equipment can be started, but only after a carefully considered plan for decontamination has been worked out. This paper describes many of the methods, equipment, and materials used for decontamination, together with the reasons why some methods work better than others for a given set of circumstances.

General

Radioactive contamination, sometimes referred to as radioactive dirt, is normally held onto a surface either chemically or physically, or by a combination of both mechanisms (1). Chemically held contamination usually adheres to the surface by means of a chemical combination with the substrate or with an oxide or other chemical compound formed by the substrate. Physically held contamination is held either by electrostatic charges or by occlusion or inclusion in the pores, cracks, or holes in the surface, or by greases or oxides on the

*Work done under the auspices of the U.S. Atomic Energy Commission.

surface. The problem of removing these contaminants from the surface may be easy and a vacuum cleaner may suffice, or they may be held so tightly that a layer of the surface must be removed in order to effect the decontamination.

Cleanliness is a relative term. After the cleaners have scrubbed and waxed our office floors, there is no visible loose dirt present. However, no one would eat food that had accidentally been dropped on the "clean floor." We regard the dinner dishes as being washed clean; however, one could not use these same dishes to grow cultures in a bacteriological laboratory. We can sterilize petri dishes to a point where they are satisfactory for growing cultures, but radioactive contamination could still be present in rather large and hazardous amounts. Thus, what may seem clean to our secretary and to the bacteriologist may not be radioactively clean. It is only after the radiation levels have been brought down to acceptable health levels that the area can be reused. If tracer experiments are to be conducted, considerations of radiation backgrounds will require levels far below those of significance from the health physics point of view.

Special Problems in Connection with Radioactive Decontamination

In ordinary circumstances, the janitor sweeps the room floor, picks up the dirt in a dust pan, and puts the refuse in a trash can for disposal. He dusts the furniture, washes areas that are particularly soiled, and does whatever needs to be done without any special precautions. The dusts which he breathes are not usually toxic, and there are no exposure problems involved. On the other hand, if he is cleaning a room that is grossly contaminated with radioactive material, he must take many precautions. He must wear protective respiratory equipment to keep the radioactive dust from entering his body. He must be cautious regarding exposure to radiation from the dirt adhering to surfaces in the area. He must wear a specially designated uniform that will be washed under controlled conditions. The operation must be monitored frequently to evaluate the exposures received by the workers and to determine how well the "clean-up" is progressing.

Another extremely important problem in radioactive decontamination is that of redeposition of the material. As the contamination is removed from a surface onto the sponge, brush, scrubber, or into a solvent, the latter must not be allowed to come in contact with cleaner areas, as the contamination picked up will in turn contaminate another surface. Since many decontaminating solutions are electrolytes, a number of the metal ions being carried by the acid tend to attach themselves tightly to other surfaces. Radioactive isotopes of cobalt, zirconium, cesium, ruthenium, and copper, for example, are notorious for redepositing on other surfaces if not removed from the environment in each successive cleaning operation. While these radioactive nuclides may be removed from the surface and taken into solution, there is a strong driving force, much like that used in electrolytic plating, to redeposit them on clean metal. This tendency can be lessened by the addition of redeposition retardants which are often found in laundry compounds, such as methylcellulose, ethylcellulose, carboxymethylcellulose, and protein complexes. Complexing agents for preventing metal ions from redepositing on metal surfaces work best when in acidic solutions.

A good example of cross-contamination or recontamination can be observed in the laundering of contaminated protective clothing. If a "clean" garment is washed in the same wash with contaminated garments, the "clean" garment will come out of the wash with some measurable contamination. The radioactive substance is dissolved or picked up by the water, and some of it is deposited in the clean garment. It should also be pointed out that any garment which has been contaminated will always contain some residual contamination.

Decontamination of Small Areas Vs. Large Areas

If a laboratory technician spills even an appreciable amount of radioactive liquid in a fume hood, the problem of decontamination is relatively simple. If it is apparent that the spill has taken place, and he realizes that he has contamination in this confined area, he closes the hood door to prevent its spread into the laboratory. He consults other workers who have had experience in such cleanup work and proceeds to collect all equipment and supplies necessary to do the job in an orderly fashion. By knowing the isotope, he can choose a cleaning material which will probably be most effective. By knowing the type of surface, he will know whether to use chemical or mechanical methods for doing the work. By knowing the method of deposition of the radionuclide on the surface, the temperature during and after deposition, and the time of residence of the material on the surface, he will have information as to the difficulty of removing the contamination. He can bring in special waste containers for safe storage of the radioactive waste. His big concern now is to prevent undue radiation exposures to the people doing the work. After the area has been cleaned to the point where there is no visible contamination, it is resurveyed for evidence of radioactivity to determine whether more cleaning is required. If the radioactivity has not been reduced to acceptable levels, the same procedure must be repeated, perhaps with stronger decontaminating agents. In case the contamination levels cannot be reduced sufficiently, it may be necessary to remove the floor or other portions of the hood for disposal. In many cases these hood parts, or other apparatus which has been contaminated, can best be cleaned by removal to another area where sandblasting or chemical means can be used.

If a similar spill had occurred on a bench top or on the floor of the same laboratory, the consequences might be much more serious. The radioactivity in the spill may become airborne as it dries, and can be spread around the laboratories where the accident happened or could conceivably get into the air conditioning system and there be carried to other parts of the building. If the accident is not noticed promptly, contamination can be tracked all over the laboratory and into other parts of the building.

Ordinarily, the person involved should call for help promptly. The area should be sealed off, if possible, to prevent the spread of contamination. If airborne contamination is likely, all workers in the laboratory should be evacuated; those who will do the cleanup should wear respiratory protection. Full protective clothing, including shoe covers and gloves, should also be used since some spread of contamination is likely. When the method of decontamination has been chosen, the workers proceed to remove the contamination in very much the manner mentioned above. Radiation surveys are made at each stage of the cleanup to obtain an understanding of the progress being made. When the radioactive contamination on exposed surfaces has been cleaned to acceptable levels and the loose contamination as shown by a smear survey is insignificant, the laboratory can be put back into operation. It should be borne in mind that it is very difficult to restore an area which has been grossly contaminated, to its original condition. The residual contamination must be brought to a level which represents no health hazard. In some cases where the experiments undertaken in a given laboratory require immaculate facilities, it may be necessary following a radiation accident to remove bench tops, floor coverings, furniture parts, etc., and to replace them with new material.

A larger contamination accident may involve an entire floor of a building, or perhaps the whole building. If there is much contamination spread fairly uniformly over large areas, the decontamination problem becomes very complex. Evacuation should be prompt. Hoods should be left on, but precautions should be initiated to prevent intermixing of air from laboratory to laboratory and to corridors. Access to the building or floor should be limited to those who are involved in the cleanup.

If the radiation levels are high, it will probably be necessary to limit the time of work in a particular place, and to require the use of full protective clothing, shoe covers or boots, respiratory protection, etc. It is usually best to start at the point of highest contamination and to remove as much contamination as possible by a superficial cleaning, using vacuum cleaners, hosing, mopping, scrubbing, etc. This reduces the radiation levels, allowing longer working times for the persons doing the cleaning. In general, it is best to remove as much equipment, furniture, etc., from the room or area as practical to another area for decontamination.

Anything moved from the area requires complete wrapping so as to minimize the spread of contamination. Removal of the furniture, fixtures, laboratory equipment, etc., from the area prevents them from becoming further contaminated during the cleanup process and, in addition, leaves the area less cluttered. The equipment which cannot be conveniently removed should be wrapped to protect it from cross-contamination. It is usually best to start with the room ceiling and to work down, always being cautious to keep dust and splash at a minimum. As the area or building gets cleaner, the work times can be longer, until even the respiratory equipment is finally no longer necessary. When the radiation levels have decreased and reached a point at which they are no longer a health hazard, the final cleanup involves painting, refinishing furniture and floors, etc. The new paint will hold essentially all of the loose contamination and thus prevent any further spread of radioactivity.

The building may be out of service for several weeks. Such a cleanup may be very expensive in terms of labor and materials. The hazards associated with certain isotopes also govern the degree of cleanliness which must be reached in the decontamination process. Areas contaminated with plutonium, strontium-90, and radium are handled very differently from areas contaminated with sodium-24, tritium, and cesium-137. The radiotoxicity of the various radioisotopes depends on the half life, the energy and character of the radiation, the degree of selective localization in the body and the rates of elimination.

If a laboratory or building becomes grossly contaminated with a short-lived activity such as phosphorus-32 or iodine-131, one might well elect to close off the area and wait for physical decay to bring the radiation down to acceptable levels. This procedure has been followed many times, and it can be demonstrated that much time and expense have been saved by depending exclusively on radioactive decay. It may be necessary to do some painting in order to fix the residual contamination due to long-lived contaminants, but at least the big labor cost is eliminated by waiting.

It should be kept in mind that contamination is a problem to the experimenter whenever isotopes are used. Facilities should be designed to minimize decontamination if it ever is necessary. Ventilation should be provided to prevent the spread of airborne contamination from room to room. The floors, flat surfaces, bench tops and furniture should be made of materials which can be readily decontaminated. Heating systems using blowers tend to spread contamination. Electrical switches and valves should be provided locally so that it is possible to shut down promptly any equipment which may cause the spread of contamination. Emergency procedures should be written down and drills should be held periodically to insure that all workers understand what is to be done in case a radiation accident takes place.

Decontamination Procedures and Methods

If one is faced with the problem of decontamination, one must consider many factors before attempting the operation (2). He must answer the following questions:

1. What is the probability of success? If the surfaces of contaminated items are of wood, concrete, or other rough porous material, it is usually very difficult to clean them completely. It may be wise to dispose of them rather than clean them.

2) What are the economics involved? In some cases it may be more expensive to clean contaminated equipment than to replace it and pay for its disposal.

3) What risks are involved? The radiation levels and airborne problems may be such that conventional cleanup procedures are not appropriate. If the first part of the work requires remote-handling equipment and such equipment is not available, the material will have to be stored safely or disposed of.

4) Will the usual decontaminating agents be effective on the material to be decontaminated? This will help to determine which, if any, decontaminant will be used.

5) How about the heat resistance of the material to be cleaned? Some materials tend to deform even at relatively low temperatures, precluding the use of hot decontaminating solutions.

There are two principal methods of wet decontamination: total immersion and the "piecemeal" method. Immersion is applicable primarily to equipment that can actually be covered by a decontaminating liquid. Figure IV-1 shows a stainless steel tank facility equipped with heat, water, and steam. The cleaning solution can be heated, and the various processes of decontamination such as diffusion, ion exchange, or chemical action can effectively work on the item to be cleaned. After soaking or scrubbing, the item can be rinsed in a tank of clean solution, dried, and monitored. If the levels of contamination are still too high, the equipment can be treated again. The advantage of this method is that exposures can be kept low, since the item to be cleaned can be handled at a distance and can be soaked for as long as is necessary, without the operator's attendance. The big disadvantage of large tanks, however, is the vast amount of cleaning solutions needed to decontaminate large equipment.

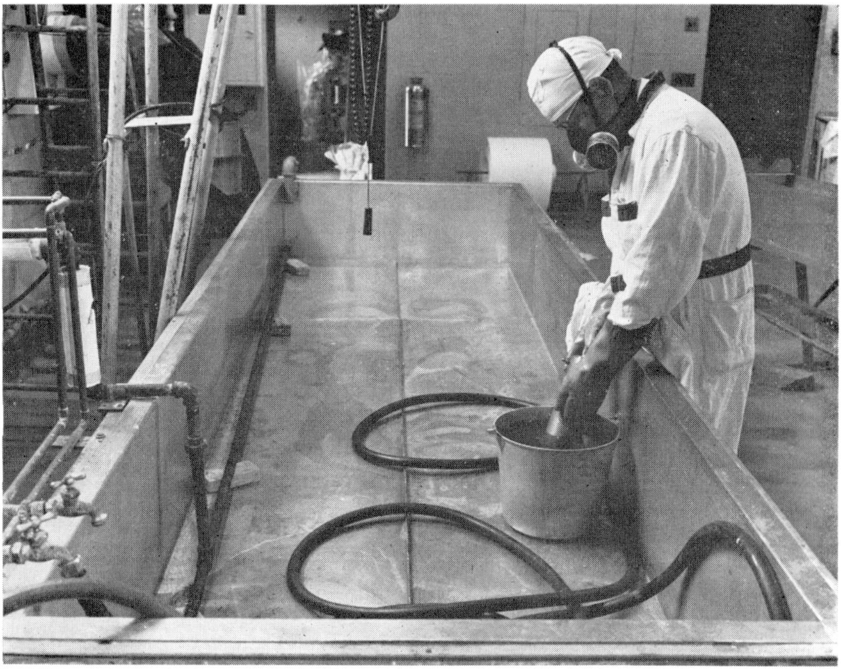

FIGURE IV-1. Large stainless steel decontamination tank, equipped with all utilities, at Brookhaven National Laboratory.

Ultrasonic devices are being used to speed up the cleaning process, but in general, these devices are used only for small articles such as instrument parts and articles with awkward, hard-to-clean shapes. Larger ultrasonic cleaners have been installed at considerable expense and have given very satisfactory results.

"Piecemeal" decontamination means the cleaning of large items a little at a time, usually by starting at the top and working down. It is always advisable to clean the "hottest spots" first so as to reduce the general radiation levels in the decontamination area. One method is to apply the decontaminating material to the item with a brush or mop, let it set for a period of time, then vigorously scrub or brush it, and finally flush it off with a clean solution. The item is then moved to another area, and the process is repeated. It may be necessary to make the decontaminating solution into a paste, especially if there are many vertical surfaces. The big advantage of this method is that it can be carried out almost anywhere, and that only small amounts of reagents are required. However, exposures of personnel tend to be much higher in "piecemeal" decontamination since longer contact times with the item are required.

Painted surfaces which have become contaminated frequently must be stripped of paint before the equipment can be cleaned satisfactorily. Stripping is usually sufficient for metallic surfaces, but it is not advisable to use this technique on porous materials such as wood or concrete as the contamination gets into the pores or grain and becomes very difficult to remove.

Decontaminating Agents and Materials

Generally, chemical decontaminating agents are classified as detergents, chelating compounds, and solvents, including both acids and alkalies. They can be mixed for special purposes, and are usually helped along by mechanical scrubbing or agitation.

At Brookhaven National Laboratory almost every "magic formula" that has appeared in the literature has been tried. Some of the cleaning materials which have worked well for others have not been effective during trials at Brookhaven. For this reason one will find a wide divergence of opinion as to what specific agents work best. The reclamation group at Brookhaven uses a large variety of materials, most of which are commercially available. A list of manufacturers of such materials can be found in the *Nucleonics* magazine's Buyers Guide (3).

In stubborn cases, acids or strong alkalies are often used. Precautions must be taken not to damage the surface excessively. Of course, the cleaning materials must be handled with care. At Brookhaven National Laboratory use is made of an inhibited phosphoric acid cleaner. It is marketed as a rust inhibitor and remover and contains an anionic detergent. It can safely be applied to most metals, and can even be used in the laundry as a "booster" cleaner. It is effective as a "piecemeal" cleaner especially in jelly form, and can also be used as a bath. For grease or the removal of contamination on greasy surfaces, trichlorethylene is an excellent solvent which is relatively safe to use. For lead, aluminum, rubber, plastics, and painted objects there are several commercially available materials containing special blends of acids, alkalies and special additives (3).

There are many so-called heavy detergents which work well as decontaminating agents. The usual ingredients include a surfactant (alkyl aryl sulphonate), sodium tripolyphosphate, sodium carboxymethylcellulose, EDTA (ethylene-diamine-tetraacetic acid), and a sodium carbonate or sulphate filler. Of course, the hotter the water used with these substances, the more effective it is for removing stubborn, sticky types of contamination.

Various kinds of acids of different concentrations are used for stubborn cases. For rapid attack one may use HCl with as much as 50 per cent concentration. For baths one would tend to use about 6 to 10 per cent HNO_3 and 90 to 94 per cent water. Ammonium oxalate or an oxalic acid bath has been used effectively as a soak. This is usually followed by a detergent bath and has been found effective by some decontamination laundries.

Abrasive decontaminants such as sandblasting and vapor blasting are used effectively at some sites. With vapor blasting, a decontaminating solution with a mild abrasive is directed by high-pressure guns on a contaminated surface. If the abrasive is fine and soft, there is little damage to the surface; of course, its decontamination effectiveness is low if it is so fine and soft that the surface is not abraded. Vapor blasting is ordinarily used within a closed cabinet for cleaning relatively small parts. The big advantage of vapor blasting lies in the fact that it is a wet method with little likelihood of airborne contamination.

Accidents at Brookhaven National Laboratory

Brookhaven has had a number of accidents involving radioactive contamination. Fortunately, none of the people involved have suffered any overexposure to radiation. The costs of restoration were not great in comparison with some of the accidents at other sites. However, experimental projects were held up, and the effort expended in man-hours and materials was considerable. Perhaps it would be appropriate to mention a few examples and to relate the methods used for decontamination.

In 1949, one of the staff had been asked to make a special strontium-90 source. This involved evaporating a solution containing strontium-90 onto a planchette. This had been done many times before in a fume hood without any problem. However, this time everyone was in a hurry, the concentrations of strontium in the solution were much higher, the heat source much hotter, and the work was done on a bench in the center of the room. The building heat was provided by radiators mounted on the walls, with blowers for forced-air circulation. Instead of evaporating to dryness slowly in a confined area, the solution evaporated rapidly as a mist. It was picked up by the circulating room air, and the strontium-90 was deposited in varying amounts throughout the building. Even though only a few millicuries were involved, the entire building had been contaminated, including the walls (concrete block), ceilings (sheet rock), floors (concrete), and all of the equipment. Fortunately, the operator brought his new source to a health physicist for a contamination check. It was evident immediately that the operator, as well as everything that he had touched, was grossly contaminated.

Every fixture, every piece of furniture and equipment in the building was wrapped and removed from the building for decontamination elsewhere. Many items were sent directly to a waste disposal point.

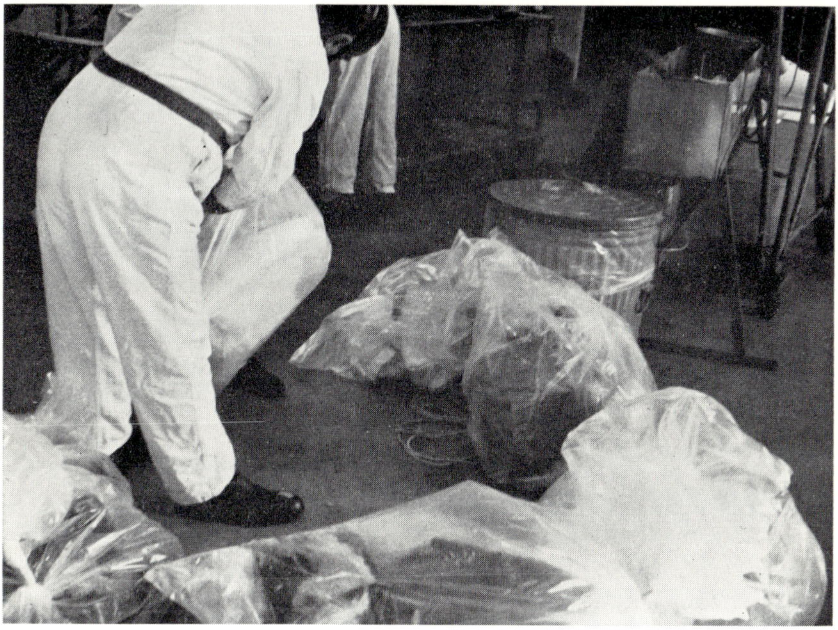

FIGURE IV-2. Decontamination facilities and packages of contaminated equipment.

(Figure IV-2 shows such a decontamination facility with contaminated material in plastic. A waste can is shown upper center, along with cleaning tanks and flexible ducting for "on the spot" ventilation.) Two-man decontaminating crews worked for weeks dismantling, sanding, and scrubbing the building. For the first four weeks, all workers were required to wear complete protective equipment including respirators. When the radiation levels had finally been reduced to acceptable limits, the entire interior of the building was painted. Continuous air samples were taken for months afterwards to determine whether the contamination had been fixed. Even to this day, fourteen years later, this building is suspect. For example, no one can enter the attic without special precautions. It is a monument to a spill, and it still requires surveillance.

Another accident involving an entire army-barrack type of building took place in 1957. One of the physicists was using a rather large phosphorus-32 source. In order for the beta particles to pass, one side of the source was protected by a thin rubber hydrochloride window. Unfortunately, this thin fragile window broke during the late afternoon and a small portion of the radioactive powder leaked out. This experiment had been in progress for several days, so that the work had become routine. Monitoring procedures for checking the source and the area had become lax and, as a result, the accident went undetected for several hours. In the meantime, the contamination had been tracked all over the building, into cars, and finally into some of the homes. Fortunately, the contaminating isotope was short-lived so that there was no great health hazard involved. Nevertheless, an attempt was made to clean up the people, cars, and homes that same night.

Since the radioactive material was essentially phosphorus-32 with only a very small amount of impurities, it was decided to remove the source for safekeeping and to close off the building completely. This was done, and at the end of five half lives, the building was restored. This period of decay was sufficient for the radiation levels to reach acceptable working conditions. The two or three most contaminated rooms were painted, and operations were resumed. Decay in this case was much the easiest way out.

A similar accident took place three years later in a similar building; this time, however, the source was 10 curies of polonium-210. Unfortunately, the accident was not detected for several days because of faulty monitoring techniques. As a result, polonium-210 was tracked to many parts of the laboratory and was carried home on shoes and clothing. Personnel were cleaned up as promptly as possible, and no one suffered any appreciable exposure. The job of decontamination took weeks. As before, all fixtures, furniture and equipment were wrapped and removed to another area for decontamination. Teams scrubbed ceilings, walls, floors, ducts, etc., for weeks. Full respiratory and protective clothing was required during the initial phases of the cleanup. When the radiation levels had reached the point where a health hazard no longer existed, all surfaces were again painted over. New linoleum was installed on the floors and new treads were placed on the stairs. The equipment was cleaned up piece by piece, repainted, and brought back to the laboratory. Radioactive decay helped in this situation, but it was believed that waiting for decay would leave the building unoccupied too long. Therefore, it was decided to proceed with the decontamination. Today, after decontamination and the passing of ten half lives, the area is used without restriction.

Decontamination of the Brookhaven National Laboratory Reactor Canal

The Brookhaven National Laboratory Research Reactor Canal, which is used to handle irradiated fuel, became grossly contaminated over the years. After the last of the irradiated natural uranium fuel had been removed, it was decided to clean up this facility. This was probably the largest and most hazardous decontamination job that had been undertaken at Brookhaven National Laboratory (4).

The poured concrete walls and floor of the canal had been painted ten years before with a vinyl paint. The canal was sixty-four feet long, six feet wide, and nine feet deep.

Before the water was drained from the part of the canal to be decontaminated, all fuel elements and all other items stored there were moved to the deep pit (Figure IV-3). A dam was installed to keep the water in the deep pit from entering the area to be cleaned. Decontamination was begun by lowering the canal water level two feet at a time, so as to expose only a narrow band of the highly contaminated wall. The water remaining in the canal was filtered con-

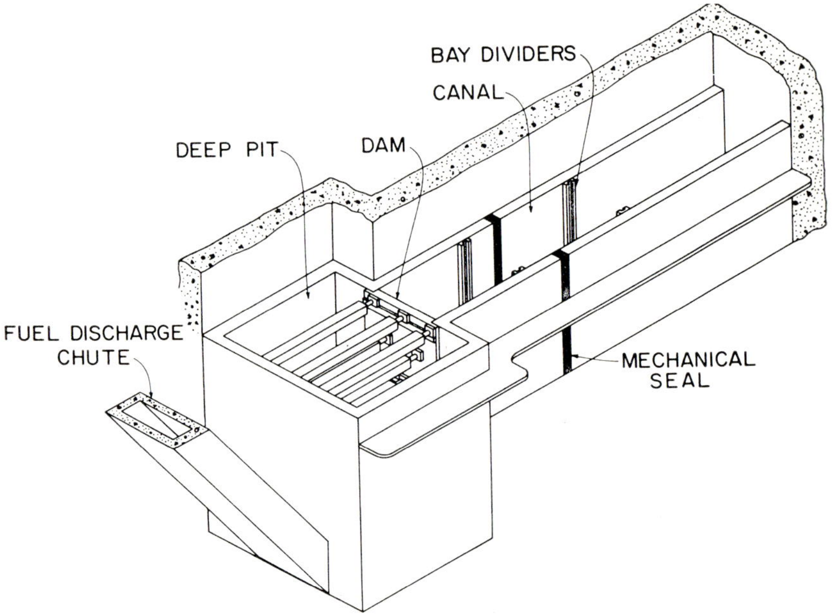

FIGURE IV-3. Drawing of Brookhaven National Laboratory's Graphite Research Reactor Canal.

tinuously to keep it as clean as possible. It acted as a shield against the radiation below the water surface. After the water had been completely drained, plywood sheets were laid on the bottom and against the side walls. This afforded some protection to the workers against excessive beta radiation. The plywood sheets were moved only enough to expose a relatively small work area. The paint from this area of concrete wall was stripped by the use of an organic coating remover. Most of the contamination came off with the paint. To remove the paint residue and to decontaminate still further, the surfaces were steam cleaned using a special cleaner which provided a quick wetting action, and a mild blend of alkaline salts and sequesterants that resulted in rapid and effective decontamination. The concrete surfaces were then etched with a de-oxidizing agent before repainting.

There were 68 men involved with this job. During certain stages, the workers wore supplied-air masks, protective clothing, gloves and boots. At other times, respirators with ultrafilters were sufficient. The crews consisted of four workers and one health physicist. These were changed frequently in order to distribute the doses as evenly as possible. In no case did any worker receive more than 300 mrem of dose during a work week. Table IV-1 shows personnel dose and working times to do the job.

Of course, there was a rather large amount of radioactive waste generated which had to be packaged and disposed of. There were many garments to be washed at the decontamination laundry, and much respiratory equipment to clean and sterilize for further use. It was a big job, but the results were very gratifying. An area that had become intolerable from the point of view of radiation safety is now relatively clean and requires only limited restrictions because of radiation.

In 1960, the new Brookhaven National Laboratory decontamination facility and decontamination laundry were completed (5). The laundry is much like any commercial one, except that radiation monitoring is part of the operation. The decontamination facility consists of a

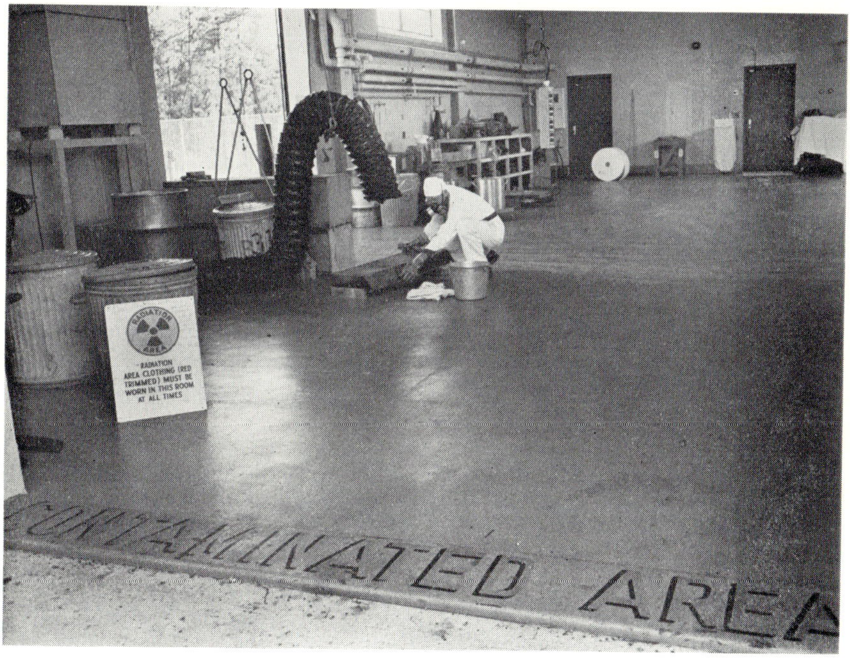

FIGURE IV-4. Interior of Brookhaven National Laboratory decontamination building, showing facilities and a sample operation.

large, uncluttered room with a smooth, easily decontaminated floor with floor drains, an overhead crane for handling large heavy objects, and an excellent filtered ventilation system (Figure IV-4). Special cleaning tanks, steam cleaning equipment, a shot blasting facility, and special movable shields are provided as tools. This facility is equipped to handle most ordinary decontamination jobs. It has been extremely useful during cleaning of large and small items from all parts of the laboratory.

Brookhaven National Laboratory's shot blasting facility was installed as part of the decontamination facility in 1962. After one year of operating experience, it is felt that this is the best method for cleaning large, bulky items with rough and porous surfaces (Figure IV-5). The Brookhaven National Laboratory facility consists of an enclosed room twelve feet wide, ten feet deep, and eight feet high, with about 22,000 cubic feet per minute of ventilation. The contaminated air surrounding the operation is filtered by two sets of bag filters

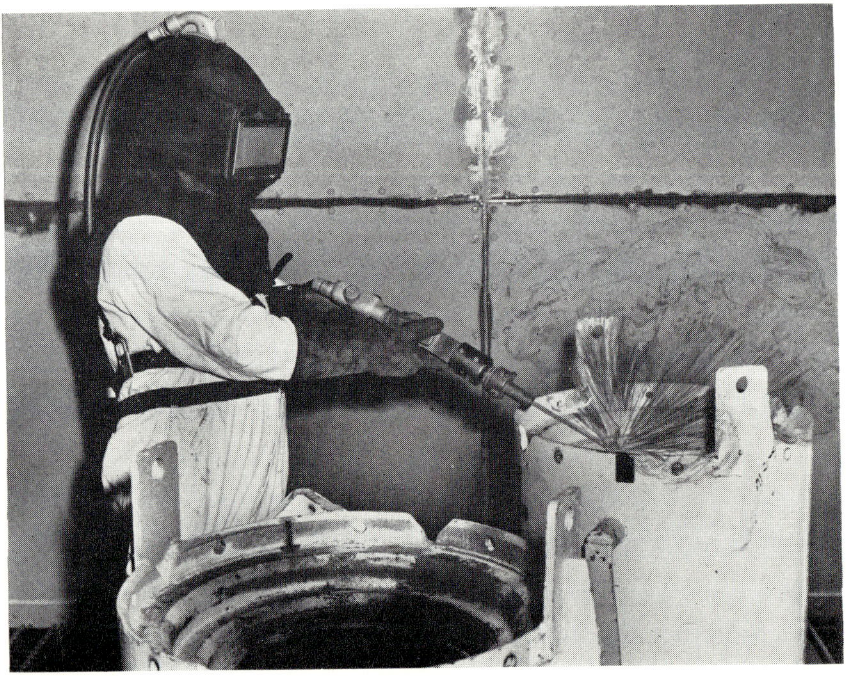

FIGURE IV-5. Decontamination by shot blasting at Brookhaven National Laboratory.

in series, followed by a bank of absolute filters. The operator is equipped with complete protective respiratory equipment and clothing. The exposure rates may be somewhat high since the operator must be in close proximity to the item being cleaned; however, the time usually required for cleaning is short, so that the exposure is often less than the more conventional means of decontamination would require.

Facilities using appreciable amounts of hazardous radioactive isotopes should have an area set aside for decontamination work (6). This does not have to be an elaborate setup, but there should be a place where contaminated items can be brought for cleaning. There is usually some low-priority space in hospitals, research institutes, or industrial plants which can be converted to a cleanup area. In the case of a hospital, it might be attached to the laundry in some way.

At the present time, there are several commercial contractors who will undertake special decontamination jobs. For small jobs, they can no doubt be effective (3). However, for the examples mentioned above, involving the strontium-90, the polonium-210, and the canal cleanup, an outside contractor would have been at a great disadvantage.

In summary, caution and common sense are the two greatest assets for doing decontamination work.

TABLE IV-1

PERSONNEL DOSE AND WORKING TIMES

	Dose in rem	*Man Days*
Dam study, fabrication, installation	0.8	14
Decontamination	3.5	12
Stripping paint	13.7	54
Sandblasting	3.4	13
Mason trowel coat	3.2	30
Painters, all coats	1.5	24
Health Physics	12.6	42
Supervision, assistance	12.9	75
Totals:	51.6	264

REFERENCES

1. Newman, Kenneth W.: Radioactive Decontaminating. *The Journal of the American Association for Contamination Control, 2*:No. 4, 15, April 1963.

2. Blythe, H. J.: *Decontamination at Harwell.* U. K. Atomic Energy Research Establishment, AERE Report 4307, 1963.
3. Decontamination—Listing of commercial companies in the United States and overseas that manufacture and sell decontaminating agents. Service companies that will perform decontamination work are also listed. *Nucleonics,* August 1963.
4. Humm, A. F., and Protter, S. R.: Reconditioning the Brookhaven Graphite Reactor Fuel Storage Canal. *Nucleonics, 21*:No. 6, 96-8, June 1963.
5. Pearsall, S. G., and Gemmell, L.: Design Features and Operational Procedures of the BNL Radiation Laundry and Reclamation Facility. *Am. Ind. Hyg. Assoc. Quarterly, 22*:3, June 1961.
6. *Civil Defense Manual for Radiological Decontamination of Municipalities,* Contract #OCD-05-62-279, OCD Subtask #3236A. Curtis Division, Curtis Wright Corp., Caldwell, New Jersey, August 1963.

PERMISSIBLE LEVELS OF SURFACE CONTAMINATION

WILLIAM R. BUSH

Radiation and Industrial Safety Branch
Atomic Energy of Canada Limited,
Chalk River, Ontario

WHY ARE WE concerned about surface contamination? We are concerned because we may be irradiated by it. How would we be irradiated? Either externally by proximity to contaminated surfaces, or internally after inhalation or ingestion of the contaminant. Operators of low-level counting laboratories are concerned for different reasons: contamination increases their background counting rate.

How much contamination is hazardous? A maximum permissible level of surface contamination is calculated by assessing the radiation hazard in relation to the maximum permissible dose recommended by the International Commission on Radiation Protection (ICRP).

Inhalation of radionuclides is often the greatest hazard associated with surface contamination, although this depends on many factors, such as the radiotoxicity of the nuclide, the geometry of contaminated surfaces, air movement, physical and chemical properties of the dust, and the dilution of the radionuclide with non-radioactive material.

The concentration of a radionuclide in the air above a contaminated surface may be estimated by using a dispersion constant which relates air contamination to surface contamination. Dispersion constants have been measured under various conditions, with results that vary by a factor of 10^4 (1, 2, 5, 12). A value often quoted is 2×10^{-8} cm^{-1}, which was measured when shovelling building rubble in open air (7). To illustrate, one MPC_a (maximum permissible concentration in air—ICRP) of strontium-90 would result from surface contamination of 10^{-2} $\mu c/cm^2$:

$$10^{-2}\ \mu c/cm^2 \times 2 \times 10^{-8}\ cm^{-1} = 2 \times 10^{-10}\ \mu c/cm^3 = 1\ MPC_a$$

Another hazard, which is considered less serious than inhalation, is *ingestion*. To evaluate ingestion, one must assume a relation between surface and skin contamination, and a value for the fraction of skin contamination transferred to the mouth. An interesting example showing how different conditions can affect the assessment of hazards is seen when one compares the British and Indian views of the ingestion hazard. The British assume that 1 to 10 per cent of hand contamination will be transferred to the mouth and ingested (2, 6, 8, 11). This is reasonable, with British living habits; as a result, they rate ingestion as less hazardous than inhalation. The Indians, however, assume that all contamination left on the hands will be ingested; consequently, they rate ingestion as a greater hazard than inhalation. Their assumption is also reasonable, under Indian living conditions, because many Indians, when eating, handle their food with bare hands. Furthermore, the food is often pasty and acts as a good decontaminating agent (11, 12).

The hazard of *external radiation* from contaminated surfaces depends on the type of radiation (alpha particle, beta particle or gamma-ray), its energy, and on the geometry of a man in relation to the contamination and to any shielding that may be present. Another factor to consider is beta-particle irradiation of contaminated skin or of skin in contact with contaminated surfaces. This could result in an appreciable beta-ray dose to the skin.

In this paper, I am going to ignore the external radiation hazard and talk more about the inhalation hazard. However, one should realize that external radiation might be the predominant hazard in some circumstances.

The amount of radioactive material which can safely be inhaled or ingested covers an enormous range. For example, the same amount of radiation injury is produced by exposure to a million times as much carbon-14 as plutonium-239 (on a curie basis). To overcome this complication, general contamination limits are based on the more radiotoxic nuclides, that is, on those with low values of MPC_a. These are usually plutonium-239, or radium-226 for alpha-particle emitters, and lead-210 or strontium-90 for beta-particle emitters. It follows that the limits might not be realistic for a user of less hazardous radioactive nuclides. Nevertheless, it is convenient to use a single standard for all radioactive nuclides, since no undue hardship is imposed during routine control of contamination if a hazard is overestimated by a factor of a million or so.

Limits applied in various countries are listed in Table IV-2. In general, those used in India are lowest, while the highest are in Britain and France. Those specified in the United States vary considerably from one establishment to another. Variations are to be expected, because the nature of the contaminant and the type of operation vary widely from one establishment to another. Even for identical operations in different countries, it is not surprising to find different limits, because some of the assumptions made in calculating the limits are quite arbitrary.

The maximum permissible levels of beta-emitting contamination at various establishments vary from 10^{-5} to 10^{-3} microcuries per square centimeter ($\mu c/cm^2$). They are frequently relaxed by a factor of 10 when applied to contamination-prone areas, and made more restrictive for normally clean areas such as offices. The limits for alpha-emitting contamination are generally ten times more restrictive than those for beta-emitting contamination, particularly if actinium, polonium, plutonium or radium is present. But no matter what value one chooses for the maximum permissible level, there will normally be no justification for leaving loose, easily removed contamination on a surface.

We do not specify numerical limits at Chalk River. Instead, we specify that there shall be no readily detectable surface contamination in most areas, and that the amount in areas most prone to contamination shall be as low as practicable. The residual contamination in most areas rarely exceeds 100 counts per minute of beta- or gamma-ray emitters (cpm β) on a smear sample (the lower limit for easy detection). The level of radioactive substances in our most contamination-prone areas rarely exceeds 5000 counts per minute (cpm). These correspond to about 5×10^{-5} and 2×10^{-3} $\mu c/cm^2$, respectively.

Our policy is easy to apply at Chalk River because we employ decontamination personnel continuously in the various operating areas. They are very busy when maintenance and repair operations are in progress and when contamination escapes from a system; however, during normal operations they have time to remove even traces of contamination from surfaces. In practice, this means that floors in contamination-prone areas are mopped, using strong detergent, about once per day.

In establishments where operating personnel do their own decontamination, or where decontamination squads are called in only when unusually high levels of contamination occur, it is good practice to specify numerical limits. Furthermore, different limits are desirable for different types of work; otherwise, contamination in areas which are relatively easy to keep clean will accumulate to levels found in contamination-prone areas. Although this would not be particularly hazardous, it would be contrary to the general philosophy of radiation protection—there shall be no unnecessary exposure.

Respirators may have to be worn when high concentrations of surface contamination are present. At what concentration should one wear a respirator?

Since the maximum permissible level of surface contamination (MPL_{SC}) is loosely related to MPC_a, the guide for wearing respirators in contaminated areas could be similar to that used for wearing them when the air contamination is known. For example, if one specified that respirators be worn when (anticipated exposure period) times (level of air contamination) exceeds one MPC_a-hour, then one could similarly specify that they be worn when (anticipated exposure period) times (surface contamination level) exceeds one MPL_{SC}-hour.

Such a rule might be a useful guide, but considerable judgment has to be used in applying it. For example, if one spent only one hour per month decontaminating surfaces, he could do so without a respirator at contamination levels much higher than would be permitted if he spent one hour per day doing the same work.

The nature of an operation might be more important than the level of contamination. Respirators should be worn during any dust-raising operation, even if the contamination level is low. For example, sweeping a contaminated floor would be more hazardous than cleaning it with a damp mop. Working in a small, crowded, contaminated area would be more hazardous than doing the same work in open air over the same level of surface contamination.

I have been discussing levels of contamination encountered during routine operations. Now, I should like to consider *emergencies* that involve unusually high levels of contamination.

Emergency actions will occasionally be taken, following contamination accidents, without use of a respirator or a radiation survey.

Although routine precautions and dose limits might be ignored, one could cope with the situation more efficiently if he had an order-of-magnitude knowledge of the degree of danger. This would require that radiation hazards be assessed *before* emergencies arise, and that areas be identified with respect to the potential degree of danger.

It is convenient to draw up a reference table of inhalation hazards from various radionuclides under certain nominal conditions, such as from one curie spread over the floor. This has been done in Table IV-3, in which the potential level of surface contamination was taken as the amount of radionuclide kept in a room, divided by an assumed floor area of 10 m^2. When multiplied by a dispersion constant, this gives the concentration in air, from which the number of MPC_a's can be calculated. To obtain a measure of the inhalation hazard, this must be multiplied by the exposure time, yielding MPC_a-hours of intake. It might be reasonable to allow one year's permissible intake to be inhaled in a single emergency exposure; that is, 2000 MPC_a-hours (40 hr/wk $\times$ 50 wk/yr). This would irradiate the critical organ with 12, 15, or 30 rem, depending which organ is critical for the nuclides involved. Even if this amount is not permitted in a single exposure, it is a useful standard with which large intakes can be evaluated.

For example, under conditions assumed in Table IV-3, one curie of strontium-90 gives 300 MPC_a. Therefore, an area would be designated as dangerous if it contained more than $\frac{2000}{300} = 7$ curies of strontium-90 (assuming an emergency exposure time of one hour). Such an area could be color-coded to identify it as potentially dangerous. If a contamination accident occurred, one would then know at a glance the maximum degree of danger to expect.

Summary

Surface contamination is undesirable because it gives rise to radiation hazards.

Inhalation hazard is often the determining factor in setting contamination limits; however, external radiation could be a greater hazard under some circumstances.

The relationship between contamination level and radiation hazard is not precise, because of wide variations in actual conditions.

Permissible levels of contamination are based on many arbitrary assumptions. When assessing dangerous levels of contamination, permissible levels should be recalculated using the best information available for all parameters.

Potentially dangerous areas should be identified with respect to the maximum degree of danger likely to be met in a contamination accident.

There are some important aspects of the contamination problem that I have not considered, such as the relative degree of hazard from inhalation and external radiation under various conditions, and the need for ventilation, filtration and containment after a contamination accident. There are many possibilities for research into such problems.

I have found the subject of surface contamination much more challenging, far-reaching and interesting than I anticipated when starting to prepare this paper. I hope I have conveyed some of this impression to you.

TABLE IV-2

MAXIMUM PERMISSIBLE LEVELS OF SURFACE CONTAMINATION (MPL_{sc})

$\mu c/cm^2$

	Alpha	*Beta*
United States	10^{-7} to 10^{-6}	10^{-5} to 10^{-4}
United Kingdom (7)	10^{-4}	10^{-3}
France (10)	10^{-4}	10^{-3}
Union of Soviet Socialist Republics (12)	6×10^{-7}	10^{-4}
International Atomic Energy Agency (9)	10^{-4}	10^{-4}
India (12)	3×10^{-6}	3×10^{-5}
Canada*	10^{-5}	10^{-3}

Notes: The limit for alpha-particle emitters is generally relaxed by a factor of ten if actinium, polonium, plutonium or radium are not present.

The limit in inactive areas is generally ten times more restrictive than in contamination-prone areas.

*Although no official limit is specified at Chalk River, these tentative limits will probably be applied at WNRE, Atomic Energy of Canada Limited's new research centre at Whiteshell, Manitoba.

TABLE IV-3

INHALATION HAZARD—MPC_a

From 1 Curie Spread Over $10 m^2$

Surface contamination = $10 \mu c/m^2$

air contamination = $10^{-7} \mu c/m^3$ (dispersion constant = $10^{-8} cm^{-1}$).

Nuclide	*No. of MPC_a (40 h)*
Pu^{239}	50,000
Ra^{226}	3,000
Au^{198}	0.5
Cs^{137}	10
I^{131}	10
Sr^{90}	300
Co^{60}	10
Ca^{45}	3
P^{32}	1
Na^{24}	10^{-4}
C^{14}	0.02

REFERENCES

1. Bailey, J. C., and Rohr, R. C.: *Airborne Contamination from Surfaces.* Oak Ridge Gaseous Diffusion Plant, Report K 1088, 1953.
2. Barnes, D. E.: *Basic Criteria in the Control of Air and Surface Contamination; Health Physics in Nuclear Installations.* Symposium at Danish Atomic Energy Centre of Riso, May 1959.
3. Barry, E. V., Eisenbud, M., and Blatz, H.: How Important is Surface Contamination? *Nucleonics, 12*:No. 8, 12, 1954.
4. Becher, A. F.: *The Development of Surface Alpha Contamination Limits.* Symposium on Occupational Health Experience and Practice in the Uranium Industry, Health and Safety Laboratory, Report HASL-58, p. 151, 1958.
5. Chamberlain, A. C., and Stanbury, G. R.: *The Hazards from Inhaled Fission Products in Rescue Operations after an Atomic Bomb Explosion.* Atomic Energy Research Establishment, Report AERE HP/R 737, 1951.
6. Dunster, H. J.: Contamination of Surfaces by Radioactive Material; The Derivation of Maximum Permissible Levels. *Atomics, 6*:233, 1955 (revised from AERE HP/R 1495).
7. Dunster, H. J.: Surface Contamination Measurements as an Index of Control of Radioactive Materials. *Health Physics, 8*:353, 1962.
8. Dunster, H. J.: *Maximum Permissible Levels of Skin Contamination.* Authority Health and Safety Branch, Harwell, Report AHSB (RP) R28, 1963.
9. Fairbairn, A.: *Notes on Certain Aspects of the Regulations.* Safety Series 7, International Atomic Energy Agency, Vienna, 1961.
10. Pomarola, J.: La decontamination des materiels et des Locaux. *Bull. Inform. Sci. et Tech., 39*:14-21, April 1960.

11. Somasundaram, S., Hariharan, P. V., and Ganguly, A. K.: *Maximum Permissible Levels of Surface Contamination.* Atomic Energy Establishment, India, Trombay, Report AEET/HP/2, 1961.
12. Venkataraman, K., *et al.:* An Evaluation of Radiation Protection Standards for Indian Conditions. *Health Physics, 9*:647, 1963.

COLD WEATHER DECONTAMINATION

JOSEPH C. MALONEY
U.S. Army Nuclear Defense Laboratory
Edgewood Arsenal, Maryland

SINCE ITS INCEPTION in 1948, the U.S. Army Nuclear Defense Laboratory, Edgewood Arsenal, Maryland, has had as one of its prime missions the study of countermeasures as applied to Army problems. Since radiation is nonselective in its effects on military and civilian personnel, the information obtained is directly applicable to the civilian population.

Radiological countermeasures taken following a contaminating event are defined as actions to achieve: a) the mission recovery, or b) productivity attendant in the occupancy of strategic areas of installations and their supporting facilities. These countermeasures comprise specially adjusted individual conduct, shielding, decontamination, and waiting for decay.

The information gained in laboratory investigations, nuclear weapon effect tests, and field tests involving radiological fallout simulants has been sorted, collated, evaluated, and published in usable form in military technical manuals. Until 1960, all the experimental work had been conducted at nuclear test sites and laboratories located in relatively warm areas; thus, information available prior to 1960 applied only to temperate weather conditions. However, since many of our permanent military installations are located in areas where cold weather conditions prevail during a significant portion of the year, a cross-service project was initiated in 1960 to collate all available pertinent cold weather information and to conduct necessary investigations under winter conditions. The bulk of the experimental work has been conducted at Camp McCoy, Wisconsin, which is approximately 250 miles northwest of Chicago. This site was selected for its optimum balance of cold weather, supporting logistics, and proximity of suitable reactor facilities for isotope supply.

Our experimental program at Camp McCoy has been basically a study of fallout decontamination procedures under winter conditions; there have also been some limited investigations of fallout migration and shielding by snow cover. The contaminant employed has consisted of radiologically tagged particles, sieved to the same particle size range, and dispersed on test surfaces at the same particle concentration as that expected in real fallout. This technique was developed by the Naval Radiological Defense Laboratory, and altered to suit our requirements.

For any contaminated built-up area, regardless of size, the same basic decontamination philosophy applies. The contaminant must be physically removed from its place of deposition and then transported to another location where its effects are innocuous to personnel. Under temperate weather conditions, the contaminant is removed from hard surfaces, i.e., roofs and pavement, by hosing or sweeping; soil areas are decontaminated by appropriate surface removal methods. However, under winter conditions the water used in hosing operations may freeze, and the frozen soil is not amenable to scraping or plowing. In addition, the contaminant may be on the top of a snow or ice cover or intermixed with it.

Winter weather can vary greatly, and there are always exceptions to rules. However, under most cold-weather conditions, the following generalizations should apply.

1) Water hoses used to decontaminate hard, bare surfaces are much less efficient than when used under temperate conditions. As the temperature drops, this method becomes marginal and finally ineffective. The hard surfaces should be decontaminated by sweeping or vacuum cleaning; municipal hopper-type street sweepers are very effective on frozen ground. They are not effective on thawed ground.

2) Contaminated surfaces covered with very light snow are best decontaminated by sweeping. Hopper-type sweepers fill up rapidly. The best approach for decontaminating large areas is to use a rotary broom, such as those used to sweep ice-skating rinks. The contaminant is swept to one side until a windrow of material is formed. Regular bulk hauling equipment would be used to transport the windrow material.

3) Deeper snow is best handled with snow-removal apparatus—

anything from hand shovels to rotary plows. Large bulldozers are especially efficient in pushing away large volumes of contaminated snow.

4) Perhaps the most difficult problem is to decontaminate ice in which the contaminant is frozen. The only solutions here are to remove the ice itself, or to melt it.

One tangible benefit of cold weather is worthy of mention—the decontamination operators, in order to stay warm, welcome lots of anti-contamination clothing as well as respirators and gas masks.

It has been our philosophy in every test to limit all decontamination methods to the utilization of equipment that can normally be found either in the road and ground maintenance departments of municipal governments and military installations, or in homes. We have made no attempt to modify any of this equipment, nor have we given the equipment operators any specific instructions as to technique, with the exception of stipulating the duration for effort studies. It is hoped that our results will accurately reflect the effectiveness which can be achieved by a worker who is experienced in the operation of a particular piece of equipment, but who has no knowledge of, or special training in, radiological decontamination.

Following this line of thought, we have also classified our decontamination results according to the type of surface. In an actual situation, the director of decontamination operations will have to decontaminate certain areas with a limited number and limited types of equipment. He will accordingly select the best available equipment and send it to the area to be decontaminated. With this in mind, our results will be given for each type of surface that was decontaminated in our studies. The two measurements reported are: a) percentage of activity remaining, and b) effort in units of man-hours per 1000 square feet. Since this is probably an unfamiliar unit to most readers, it will be related to a more familiar quantity. A street sweeper makes its rounds at an average speed of approximately five miles per hour; as a result, its unit effort level is approximately 0.015 man-hours per 1000 square feet. Effort levels will be presented as a general comparison with the street sweeper.

Packed Snow

This is the normal surface encountered on city streets after traffic has packed two to six inches of snow. Under cold conditions (less than 20°F), one pass of a mechanical sweeper will decontaminate packed snow so that 6 per cent remains. Above this temperature, the surface becomes wet, and the effectiveness of the sweeper drops to 50 per cent. In this instance, a second pass will leave 15 per cent contamination.

A mechanized vacuum sweeper will leave 15 per cent as long as the temperature is below freezing. The effort will be almost double that of a street sweeper.

Sweeping packed snow with hand corn brooms will leave 60 per cent of the activity, with an effort level nearly twenty times that of the mechanical street sweeper. Such a test was conducted very near the freezing point. It is assumed that somewhat improved decontamination efficiency can be expected at lower temperatures.

Motor grading left 15 to 20 per cent remaining after two passes at below-freezing temperatures, with an effort level equal to that of a sweeper.

Fire hosing of packed snow is feasible if the snow can be completely washed away. Under these conditions, 10 to 25 per cent remaining activity can be achieved, depending upon the temperature, the higher figure occurring near 0°F. This requires about thirty times the effort level of the sweeper. If the packed snow is not washed away, very little decontamination will be achieved.

Undisturbed Snow

A straight blade bulldozer can decontaminate loose, undisturbed snow to a level of 11 per cent remaining, at an effort level of 0.012, which is slightly less than that of the street sweeper rate. However, as the bulk of snow increases with large-area decontamination, much difficulty is encountered in controlling snow that comes off the end of the blade. This situation may require follow-up decontamination with a grader or a bucket loader.

Near the freezing point, a motor grader alone can decontaminate to a level of 5 per cent remaining, with an effort half that of the sweeper. At lower temperatures, only 35 to 45 per cent remaining can be obtained. It was observed that sand lying on top of the snow would work under the blade, thus reducing the effectiveness of the decontamination. As the snow became wet, due to higher temperatures, this effect was reduced.

The best method of loose-snow decontamination is by the use of a truck-mounted blade snow plow. The work rate is one-fifth that of a street sweeper, with 1 to 5 per cent activity remaining.

The rotary snow blower can decontaminate wet snow to 2 per cent remaining, at an effort of four times that of the street sweeper. With dry snow, there will be 15 per cent or more remaining at an effort level comparable to the street sweeper. However, this procedure causes extensive contamination downwind.

A towed pan scraper will leave 18 to 20 per cent activity, at a work rate comparable to that of a street sweeper. However, it will quickly load up with snow, and much time is consumed in hauling and dumping.

A manual self-propelled rotary snow blower will leave 8 to 35 per cent activity remaining, depending upon the temperature and the depth of snow. The effort level is high, i.e., ten times that of the street sweeper.

Small blade snow plows, either hand-pushed or self-propelled, will leave 13 and 28 per cent activity, respectively, at work rates comparable to the small rotary plow, or about ten times that of the street sweeper. The use of these small hand plows is highly dependent upon snow depth; they are impossible to use in snow depths over six inches.

The manual snow shovel will leave approximately 10 per cent activity, but, of course, with a very high effort level of two man-hours/1000 ft^2, or 135 times that of the sweeper.

Compressed air can be used, but only on thin layers of dry snow all of which can be blown away. In this case, approximately 20 per cent will remain, at an effort level triple that of the sweeper.

Bare Frozen Ground

A motor grader or dozer is ineffective on frozen ground, leaving 80 to 90 per cent of the contaminant.

A street sweeper will leave 3 to 10 per cent, depending upon the roughness of the ground. A mechanized street vacuum cleaner can also be used with comparable success.

Sweeping the ground with hand brooms will leave 25 per cent, and vacuuming with a hand vacuum cleaner, 50 per cent, both with efforts twenty times that of the mechanized street sweeper.

Compressed air can also be used on frozen ground, leaving 14 per cent at an effort ten times that of the street sweeper.

Bare Thawing Ground

As the ground begins to thaw and becomes slightly muddy, dozers, graders, and towed scrapers become effective; after two passes over the area, all leave less than 10 per cent, with effort levels of 0.050 man-hours/1000 ft^2, or triple that of the sweeper.

Approximately the same level of decontamination can be achieved by hand shovels, but with eighty times the effort.

Ice

Ice can be decontaminated with hand brooms or vacuum cleaners to 15 per cent activity remaining, with an effort thirty-five times that of the sweeper.

Other Surfaces

It has been found that, on hard, dry surfaces such as pavements and roofs, there is no temperature dependence, except with fire-hosing. With proper drainage and sufficient water supply, less than 10 per cent residual activity can be achieved at temperatures to 0°F. This is true of roofs when they are hosed from above. However, if water is lobbed from the ground, the stream breaks up into a spray and tends to freeze before it can wash the contaminant to the ground.

Summary

Table IV-4 summarizes the information presented.

In conclusion, the decontamination work of the Laboratory at Camp McCoy has produced data on the basis of which the military technical manuals on radiological decontamination can now be revised to include cold-weather planning data. The Office of Civil Defense, Department of Defense, has also supported the Camp McCoy project. Additional information has been furnished to satisfy cold-weather requirements of that Office needed for the first edition of its municipal planning and decontamination manual.

TABLE IV-4

SUMMARY OF COLD WEATHER DECONTAMINATION METHODS

Surface	*Decontamination Method*	*Contaminant Remaining in Per Cent*	*Relative Effort Level Compared with Sweeper (0.015 man-hours/1000 sq. ft.)*
Packed Snow	Mechanical Sweeper	6	1
	Vacuum Sweeper	15	2
	Hand Broom	60	20
	Motor Grader	15-20	1
	Fire Hose	10-25	30
Undisturbed Snow	Bulldozer	11	<1
	Motor Grader	5-45	1/2
	Blade Snow Plow	1-5	1/5
	Rotary Snow Plow	2-15	4-1
	Towed Scraper	20	1
	Manual Rotary Plow	8-35	10
	Manual Snow Plow	13-28	10
	Snow Shovel	10	135
	Compressed Air	20	3
Frozen Ground	Motor Grader, Bulldozer,	Ineffective	
	Mechanical Sweeper	3-10	1
	Vacuum Sweeper	12	1
	Hand Broom	25	20
	Vacuum Cleaner	50	20
	Compressed Air	14	10
Thawing Ground	Bulldozer	10	3
	Motor Grader	10	3
	Towed Scraper	10	3
	Hand Shovel	10	80
Ice	Hand Broom	15	35
	Vacuum Cleaner	15	35

WASTE GENERATION AND DISPOSAL IN EMERGENCY DECONTAMINATION

RICHARD B. O'BRIEN

General Electric Company
Nuclear Materials and Propulsion Operation
Idaho Falls, Idaho

NEARLY EVERY HUMAN activity results in the generation of waste material, much of which is potentially harmful. It has been recognized almost from the very beginning that the unwanted radioactive by-products of the atomic energy industry require special treatment in order to minimize their hazardous effects. Other segments of the industrial and social community have not been so quick to recognize their responsibilities to mankind, a fact that is evidenced by the current furor over the control of air pollution in our more densely populated areas; the controversy over pesticides; and the growing concern about the pollution of our rivers, streams, and coastal waters.

Those of us who work with atomic energy are familiar with the elaborate procedures and tight controls which have been established for the disposal of radioactive wastes. We can assert that, with the exception of nuclear weapons testing, our industry has met the challenge of maintaining a relatively contamination-free environment. Unfortunately, we have very little to be smug about. Even our normal safety programs, and specifically our routine waste handling and disposal activities, are still far too costly in terms of both dollars and manpower. When we consider the increased magnitude of the waste disposal problems arising from a serious radiation emergency, not much imagination is required to foresee that their solution could be one of the most expensive, hazardous, and time-consuming aspects of the entire incident.

Most minor accidents involving radioactive contamination are of relatively little consequence from the standpoint of the generation and disposal of contaminated wastes. In these incidents, the normal, well established waste disposal channels can be utilized with little or no modification. Of greatest concern are the accidents of low probability which result in the uncontrolled dispersal of large quantities of radioactive materials. In order to qualify for this accident category, at least three essential ingredients must combine. First, a potentially hazardous quantity of radioactive material must be present; second, the containment barriers for this material must be breached; and third, a mechanism for the dispersal of the radioactive material to normally uncontaminated areas must exist. The potential for combination of these ingredients has, of course, been recognized in connection with nuclear reactors, but it also exists in varying degrees in other plants and processes. Assuming that such a major accident has occurred and that the appropriate post-accident emergency measures have been carried out, let us look at some of the more important aspects of the recovery and waste disposal operations to follow.

Goals of the Recovery Effort

A comprehensive series of preliminary investigations and decisions must be made before the proper course of the recovery effort is charted and the magnitude of the waste disposal problem is defined. The purposes of these evaluations are:

1) To estimate the post-accident condition of the plant and its environment.

2) To determine the requirements for the preservation and recovery of data.

3) To determine the goals of the recovery operation itself. Perhaps these points warrant a little further discussion.

1) ***Condition of the Plant.*** In order to provide enough information for post-incident recovery planning, the condition of the plant must be determined as completely as possible under the existing conditions. The questions to be answered are: what is the contaminating material and what are its radiological characteristics; what is the extent of the contaminated area; what are the physical and chemical characteristics of the material; how much mechanical and structural damage was sustained; and, what are the radiological hazards in the areas where work must be done?

2) ***Data Requirements.*** Decisions also must be made as to the need for preservation and collection of evidence. If the cause of the accident is not known, data collected during cleanup may provide the sole means for arriving at a conclusion. Even if the cause is known prior to the recovery, it may be deemed desirable to obtain information on the behavior of the system itself, and of the radioactive materials released, for the benefit of the industry. These considerations have a profound effect upon the course of the recovery work and the disposition of waste material.

3) ***Goals of the Recovery Operation.*** Once the foregoing information and decisions are available, the ultimate goals of the recovery operation can be determined. If feasible, the plant may be completely decontaminated and returned to normal service. On the other hand, if the characteristics of the plant and contaminant are such that cleanup does not appear to be feasible, or if extensive physical damage has occurred, it may be decided that no further use will be made of the affected portion of the plant. These two extremes define a broad spectrum of possibilities and, in most cases, the recovery effort will probably be aimed at some intermediate goal.

The Waste Disposal Problem

Once the objectives have been fairly well established, the planning of the recovery and waste disposal operation can begin. Of importance are: estimating the volume and radioactivity of materials and equipment which will be discarded without cleaning; the decontamination methods to be used; the resulting volume, form, and activity of the waste products; and the possible alternatives for ultimate disposal.

1) ***Disposal of Materials and Equipment.*** Unfortunately, most plant areas which are susceptible to contamination in an emergency also contain complex surfaces, equipment, and systems which would be very difficult and expensive to clean. The value of such equipment must be weighed against the expense and hazard of rehabilitation, in order to determine whether to discard or retain it. In fact, these same considerations may be extended to all or a portion of the building structure itself. The amount of equipment and material to be discarded will essentially determine the volume of dry waste to be handled.

2) ***Decontamination Methods.*** The decontamination method or methods to be used should be determined, and the approximate contamination level and extent of the areas to be cleaned should be estimated. From this information, the requirements for the handling and disposal of decontamination wastes can be estimated. In most cases, manual removal of debris, followed by vacuum cleaning, should be used for initial decontamination, in order to remove and confine the bulk of the active material and thereby reduce as much as possible the external radiation hazard in the work area. The final cleaning then can be accomplished by appropriate washing, detergent scrubbing, steam cleaning, abrasion, or by whatever means is best suited to the specific job at hand. Depending on the methods and the areas to be cleaned, a considerable variation in form, volume, and radioactivity of the waste products is possible.

3) ***Waste Disposal Alternatives.*** When reasonable estimates of the volumes, forms and activities of each type of waste to be generated are available, various possible disposal methods can be investigated. The capabilities of the normal process waste disposal channels should, of course, be considered, but it is unlikely that these will prove to be of great assistance. Because of the extreme difficulty in preparing and transporting large volumes of highly contaminated material, it is probable that on-site disposal will prove to be the most attractive in a number of cases. This possibility, however, poses a problem for those installations that are not located on government reservations. During the site selection process for licensed facilities, a given site may be found suitable for the disposal of normal process wastes, but this does not mean that it would be suitable for long-term burial of wastes from a serious accident. This question of suitability is so completely dependent upon the characteristics of the site and of the waste to be stored that it is beyond the scope of this discussion. Of course, other alternatives may be developed. Specially shielded containers could be built for the transportation of waste to established, remote disposal areas, or permanent shielded storage structures could be built on-site.

One interesting possibility is that of utilizing the containment vessel of a nuclear power plant for semi-permanent storage. That is, if rehabilitation is not considered feasible, the containment vessel would merely be sealed up, with no interior decontamination at all. For incidents in the range of the so-called "maximum credible accident," this may be the *only* reasonable approach. Additional shielding would, in most cases, be required on the outside of the containment vessel in order to permit continued use of the adjacent facilities.

Waste Generation and Disposal in the SL-1* Recovery

About five months after the SL-1 accident, a contract was let by the U.S. Atomic Energy Commission to the General Electric Company to perform the remaining recovery work (1, 2). Prior to this time, the program had accomplished the recovery of victims and the determination of the status of the reactor core. The goals established for the final recovery phase were:

a) To gather and evaluate data leading to an explanation of the cause of the accident.

b) To remove the reactor core for examination and disposal.

c) To dismantle and dispose of the reactor building.

d) To decontaminate the remaining buildings and area for future beneficial occupancy.

As reactor accidents go, this was a relatively small one. The fission product inventory was generated in about 950 megawatt-days of operation over a period of two years. The magnitude of the excursion was only about 130 megawatt-seconds. Between 5 and 10 per cent of the fission product inventory was released from the pressure vessel. After five months' decay, it was estimated that between 3,000 and 4,000 curies of fission products were distributed as contamination throughout the reactor building and its environs. Mechanical damage to the reactor, pressure vessel, and overhead portions of the reactor room was rather severe. This was the result of a water hammer within the pressure vessel, which had expelled loose components from the top of the vessel and caused the vessel itself to jump upward a distance of nine feet.

The reactor building was a cylindrical steel structure, thirty-eight feet in diameter and three stories high. Initial decontamination activities were hampered because of the extremely close quarters in the reactor room, which was crowded with process equipment, shield

*Stationary Low Power Plant, National Reactor Testing Station, Idaho Falls, Idaho.

blocks, and a large quantity of debris, hand tools, and extraneous portable equipment which had to be removed and sifted for evidence. Anything that could yield valuable data, including debris, vacuum cleanings, and the entire pressure vessel and core were removed, packaged, and transported to a remote handling facility about thirty-five miles away for investigation prior to disposal. The remainder of the building was dismantled and disposed of in a locally prepared burial site rather than at the regular National Reactor Testing Station burial ground, which was some distance away over public highways. Including a layer of contaminated earth removed from the site, a total of about 80,000 cubic feet of contaminated waste was buried. The remaining buildings were decontaminated and returned to normal service. During the earlier phases of the recovery, high-level contamination was tracked throughout the main support building and reactor control room, so that the cleaning of this area was a major operation in itself.

The total job was completed in a year's time. While the recorded cost was in the range of $1,000,000, this is not truly indicative of the total costs, since a great number of volunteer workers were available from the U.S. Atomic Energy Commission's Idaho Operations Office and the U.S. Army. During the work, about 475 individuals made a total of 3240 entries into the SL-1 area and spent a total of 9325 man-hours in a radiation environment. They received a cumulative total dose of about 3480 rads to the skin and 998 rem to the whole body while performing this work. It has been estimated that the use of a local waste disposal site, rather than the normal National Reactor Testing Station burial ground, saved more than 300 man-rem of exposure. This saving resulted from the fact that the scrap materials did not have to be reduced in size and packaged for transport.

Conclusion

As the foregoing discussions and the SL-1 experience indicate, the waste generation and disposal aspects of the recovery from a severe radiation emergency may be not only expensive and time consuming, but can also result in a relatively high radiation dosage to a large number of individuals. We can do very little to change this, but a few helpful possibilities do suggest themselves. Pre-accident emergency planning can be carried to the point of estimating the magnitude of the cleanup problem for a postulated reference event and developing possible solutions to the problem of final disposition of the waste products. Such pre-planning should, of course, include provisions for minimizing the spread of contamination as much as possible during the immediate post-incident emergency phase. In the operation of a plant, continuous attention to good housekeeping and the elimination of all unnecessary equipment in areas susceptible to contamination might, in some cases, prove to be extremely helpful in minimizing post-incident waste problems. Perhaps the biggest gains to be made are in the design of new plants. We recognize the possibility of accidents by providing containment and other engineered safeguards to control the release of radioactivity to the environment. It seems logical, then, to design the interiors of these plants so that the possibility of contamination of expensive equipment is minimized and so that the decontamination of structural surfaces is made as easy as practical considerations permit. While this may not make it possible to rehabilitate a plant after an extreme accident of the maximum credible accident (MCA) class, it may result in considerable savings after an accident of lesser severity.

REFERENCES

1. *Final Report of SL-1 Recovery Operation, May 1961 thru July 1962.* Aircraft Nuclear Propulsion Dept., General Electric Company, Idaho, Report TM 62-7-704, IDO 19311, July 27, 1962.
2. *Additional Analysis of SL-1 Excursion, July thru October 1962.* Flight Propulsion Laboratory Dept., General Electric Company, Idaho, Report TM 62-11-707, IDO 19313, November 21, 1962.

DISCUSSION

Dr. L. H. Lanzl: I direct my question to Mr. O'Brien. In the process of cleaning up in an emergency, do you have a different approach when you find there are living victims? Another question which one might pose in an accident such as the SL-1 is: what is the best, fastest way to determine whether or not the persons are still alive, so that you know which method of cleanup to pursue?

Mr. R. B. O'Brien: Let me say that I don't consider myself the best qualified to answer these questions, because I was not responsible for the decisions made in the immediate post-incident emergency phase of the SL-1 accident. However, I was on the scene during part of this time.

There were significant differences in the activities carried out before we knew that the victims were dead and afterwards. After it was learned that the victims were no longer living, the pace slowed down drastically, and the remaining recovery effort was made as much as possible by remote means. You have to realize, of course, that radiation levels at that time were about 1000 R per hour in the reactor room where the victims were.

Regarding the question as to how do you know whether people are alive or not, I cannot answer that. The way it was found out here was that rescue personnel actually made penetrations into the reactor room and brought out one man who, at that time, was thought to be alive. If he was, he didn't live long. These particular people all had had enough physical injury to have caused their death, so that radiation exposure was not really a consideration. The fastest way to find out whether a man is alive or not is to go and look at him, and if you cannot tell, you had better bring him out so that a physician can look at him; or it may be necessary to send a physician in to examine him.

Mr. A. A. Weintraub (U.S. Atomic Energy Commission, Health and Safety Laboratory, New York): I have a question for Mr. Maloney in reference to the cold-weather operations. It seems that there was a lot of heavy equipment which was being used in this set of experiments, which would itself have become contaminated. I wonder whether you had any policy on this equipment—whether you just left it that way and kept using it, or whether you had to clean that up, also?

Mr. J. C. Maloney: The experience we had was that the contamination of equipment was a minor problem. In most cases, if there was a little bit of residual contamination, we just parked the equipment and waited for radioactive decay to eliminate it. There were some items such as a snow plow and front loaders which we borrowed from the camp, and at the end of the day's work, we decontaminated these machines either with brooms or with hoses or a steam cleaner. The machines were checked by the health physicist and, in every case, were found to be free of contamination.

Mr. A. A. Weintraub: Did you have any problems with your detection instruments working?

Mr. J. C. Maloney: No, they all worked well. We had a good supply of batteries. However, the instrumentation we used for taking scientific data was housed in a heated trailer, and only the detector head was out in the cold. We found that, the colder it was, the better the instruments worked.

Dr. L. H. Lanzl: I would like to direct this question to Mr. Gemmell. When is it practical to cover up the radioactivity rather than to decontaminate? I know that you have touched on this. I wonder whether you could expand on it a little.

Mr. L. Gemmell: The longer you have to work on a contaminated item, the greater is the expense to get the level down to the point where it is no longer a health hazard, and of course that level is considerably higher than the levels which you may be required to reach in tracer experiments or in low-level counting rooms. I would not care to state any magic figure, but if it is in an area where people work all the time, you should probably get the contamination level down so that a forty-hour-week accumulated exposure in the area would not be more than, shall we say, 20 to 30 per cent of the exposure limit in use. I'm sure there are people in the audience who would disagree with this, but the further you drive it down, the more expensive it becomes.

When you get to the point where you can live with the radiation level, you stop your decontamination effort and paint the contaminated surface. That is what most people do, I believe. It would be nice to get the equipment completely clean, but sometimes this is a very long and troublesome procedure.

Chairman W. S. Moos (University of Illinois): It appeared to me that, during the previous session, there was some disagreement as to what should be the correct procedures for handling casualties coming into a hospital—what has priority as to who should be treated first, or what precautions should be taken as far as decontamination is concerned. I wonder whether it would be appropriate for a group of people who are experts in this field to get together and study the problem and then make suggestions for what is the right way of doing it, and, if possible, set priorities. I don't want to start a big discussion now; I just want to bring this up as a subject.

Chapter V

SPECIFIC PROBLEMS

PROBLEMS IN HANDLING RADIUM ACCIDENTS AND EMERGENCIES

THEODORE FIELDS

Health Physics Associates
Highland Park, Illinois

THERE IS an awareness of the existence of radium exposures and contamination in all institutions using this material. The extension of regulations covering radioactivity, like those established by the U.S. Atomic Energy Commission, to the users in those states which have taken over the Atomic Energy Commission's health protection functions has swung from complete absence of control to rigid control in many states.

I shall concentrate on those medical specialties and installations which present the greatest radium problems, namely, dermatologists, radiologists, and hospitals. Current recommendations for radium storage, leak and wipe tests, record keeping, surveying and decontamination, and personnel monitoring applicable to the everyday usage of radium will be outlined. A few typical cases will be presented.

It may be well to repeat the definition of a radium accident given by Saenger (1), which is as follows: "A radium accident may be defined as an unforeseen occurrence, either actual or suspected, involving exposure of or contamination on or within humans and the environment by ionizing radiation." This type of accident is seen in those states which have now assumed the U.S. Atomic Energy Commission's health physics activities and are presently surveying the facilities for housing radium banks, storage facilities, etc.

A radium contamination may have existed unknown for many years and may not have occurred within a relatively short time before discovery. The problems arising can be air contamination, surface contamination, water contamination, or, of course, personnel contamination.

In order to determine whether a radiation emergency or accident exists, we use maximum permissible dose levels and the maximum permissible concentration levels for radium and its daughters as reference points. This sounds quite simple, but is difficult to apply in practice. For instance, when one surveys for contamination in a radium installation, it is difficult to say whether only radium-226 exists or whether all of the daughter products are being measured. (One of the daughters, lead-210 [radium D], a gamma emitter, is found in many contaminated areas; it is known to diffuse slowly through platinum and silver.) We cannot, then, use any specific values as they are stated, for instance, in Handbook #69 (2).

As an example of the difficulties encountered, let us consider the radionuclide radium-226, and the organs that may concentrate it, such as bone. If we consider a soluble compound of radium-226, the maximum permissible total-body burden would be 0.1 microcurie. The maximum permissible concentration (MPC) in drinking water used during a typical forty-hour week by controlled occupational personnel would be 0.4 picocuries (4×10^{-13} curies) per ml. The MPC for air would be 3×10^{-5} picocuries (3×10^{-17} curies) per ml. For a 168-hour-week exposure of occupational personnel, we would have a MPC for bone of 0.1 picocuries per ml. for water and 10^{-5} picocuries per ml. for air. For the total body, soluble radium-226 would give limiting values of 0.6 picocuries per ml. for water for forty hours and 5×10^{-11} microcuries per ml. for air, etc.

It is very difficult to keep all of these figures in mind during a survey. In addition, it is nearly impossible to get any definite ideas as to what radionuclide is being measured. Therefore, the safest approximation is to assume that all of the possible daughter nuclides which might exist are present. In this case, we would refer to Table IV in Handbook #69 which advises that, if radium-226 is present, the continuous occupational exposure level for a 168-hour week should not be greater than 4×10^{-13} microcuries per ml. On the other hand, if we use Table III in Handbook #69, the value for continuous exposures when radium-226 and -228 are present should not be greater than 10^{-6} microcuries per ml. of water. In any case, the continuous occupation level of water intake should not be greater than 10^{-7} microcuries per ml. These, then, are the applicable MPC values for water and air.

For the purpose of making surveys and protecting personnel, we still have to establish a level above which contamination is considered to be present, and above which a problem exists. We can extrapolate from the MPC's for beta-particle emitter contamination, using the figure of 1000 counts per minute from a two-square-inch area measured with a 30 milligram per cm^2 Geiger-Mueller counter on contact. Assuming an RBE of 20 for alpha particles, it would take fifty alpha-particle counts per minute from an equal two-square-inch area, using an alpha-particle counter, to produce a contamination level which is biologically comparable to the 1000-beta-particle count per minute. This value turns out in practice to be near 400 counts per minute for a 100-square-centimeter area when measured with an alpha-particle proportional or scintillation counter. We have described this value in terms of counts per minute rather than disintegrations per minute. It may be close to 1000 disintegrations per minute over a 100-square-centimeter area. Saenger (1) states that the Taft Public Health Center recommends 150 disintegrations per minute for a 100-square-centimeter area as the maximum level of contamination for alpha particles, which means about 1.5 disintegrations per minute per square centimeter. This seems like a very low value. It is a rate often found on the surface of a new lead brick. One would hesitate to try to decontaminate a solid piece of lead. One thousand disintegrations per minute per 100 square centimeters may be a more practical maximum level to use when one is decontaminating an area.

In any event, there is a need for setting a very definite as well as reasonable alpha-particle decontamination level. Certainly, the value of zero is not practical. One can rarely decontaminate to more than 98 per cent or 99 per cent of the original level.

Radium sources are available in a variety of designs. The needle type is a pointed hollow tube, with an eye for thread at the opposite end. The radium is sealed within the tube and forms a permanent needle. There is also the sheathed needle, which is designed so that the tip may be unscrewed. The sealed radium is contained in a platinum cell which can be removed from the hollow needle. The total filtration of these needles is usually equal to about 0.5 millimeter of platinum. The sheathed needles may have different lengths, and can hold platinum cells with different amounts of radium, thus providing a very flexible treatment system. The sheathed needle can also be used with radon tubes.

Tubes are available which are similar to needles, except that they are rounded on both ends. Tubes usually are made of a 1.0 or 0.5 millimeter thick platinum-iridium alloy which is harder than platinum and more rugged. They are constructed so that one end is removable by unscrewing. Radium can be placed in the tubes in the form of cells or needles.

Plaques present the most difficult radium contamination problems. They are flat, hollow applicators having one face, usually made of thin monel metal, about 0.5 millimeter thick. On that surface a layer of radium-226 is permanently plated. Plaques can be obtained in many sizes, usually of 5 to 10 milligrams maximum strength. Filters are added to the radium layer to remove the beta radiation and, in some instances, to "harden" the gamma radiation. Plaques are used chiefly for the treatment of superficial skin lesions.

Some recommendations are presented here for reducing the likelihood of incidents and accidents which may arise in the handling of radium.

Accountability. Wherever radium or radon are used, there must be a person who has custody of these sources. There must be an area in which they can be held safely. The person in charge must keep permanent records of the issue and return of the radium or radon. The records should, as a minimum, include the following: a) the date of the order for the source and the date issued; b) the patient, hospital, department, and/or physician who issues the order; c) the type of radium or radon used, the absolute identity of the particular source, and its total number of milligrams or radioactivity; d) the name of the person to whom the radium or radon was issued, and the signature of the person who received the material, with the date and time of issue; and e) the date of expected return, and the actual date of return of the material, with the signature of the responsible officer certifying the return and inspection of the sources.

There should be a periodic inventory of all the radioactive sources by the person in charge of the supply, in order that the books may be balanced.

Protection Surveys. A survey must be made of every facility which is used for the handling or storage of radium or radon, including all storage containers, carriers, and shields. The survey should be made under the supervision of a qualified expert, and in accordance with the recommendations of *Handbook #73* (4).

Areas used for preparing radium applicators should be routinely monitored for alpha-particle emitter contamination.

Radium Leakage. All radium sources should be tested for contamination upon receipt. If there is reason to believe that a source has been damaged, that source must be inspected. All sources should be tested routinely for leaks at intervals not exceeding one year, and preferably every six months. If testing facilities are not available locally, arrangements for the test must be made with a qualified laboratory. There are two types of tests which can be performed; each has its merits. One is a technique in which activated charcoal is placed in a container with water. The radium source is immersed in the water and charcoal for twenty-four hours (3). The other method is to use a container in which the source is placed and covered with cotton or filter paper. The source is sealed in the container for at least one day. In both methods, counts of the surrounding medium are made with a scintillation well counter on the day after the sources have been removed. Contamination levels or leakage levels are then derived by standard methods.

Personnel Monitoring Devices. These devices are required for each individual if there is a reasonable possibility of an exposure exceeding 1.25 roentgens. This limit excludes therapeutic or medical exposures. It is recommended that all persons making therapeutic use of radium routinely wear film badges. Before a person is allowed to handle radium, he must be informed of the hazards involved and how to guard against them. Everybody handling radium must read and understand *Handbook #73* (4) and the U.S. Department of Health, Education and Welfare Guide for Protection Against Radiation from Radium.

In every hospital, clinic, or laboratory handling radium, there should be a radiation safety officer with the necessary authority to carry out and enforce the directives of a radiation safety committee. He must be directly responsible for working conditions which conform to the current standards of the pertinent guides and to federal, state, and local regulations. He should have available one or more portable instruments capable of detecting gamma radiation levels as low as 0.1 milliroentgen per hour.

For purposes of illustration, we can consider several types of radiation accidents. The low-level, prolonged type of radium contamination incident is typically found in a dermatologist's office after the break of a radium plaque. Since the age of most of these plaques is about ten to twenty years, such contamination could have been present for several years. Both internal and external radium exposures may be caused in this way.

Excessive brief radium exposure demands immediate consideration. It may occur when a radium needle is broken in transit, or perhaps upon its delivery to a medical office or hospital. The exposure in this case may be from external gamma radiation as well as from inhalation or ingestion of the subsequent contamination.

Excessive prolonged radium exposure quite often occurs where radium sources have been stored with very little shielding, for example, without lead bricks or with inadequate amounts of lead. In addition, it is quite possible to have a large amount of radium or radon leakage from the radium needles themselves.

Certain equipment and supplies are necessary if any of the three types of incidents noted above occurs. They must be available to each health physicist who intends to do any kind of decontaminating or surveying work in a radium installation. The extent of their use depends on the levels of contamination or exposure found:

A) A pocket alarm type Geiger-Mueller counter (the pocket "Chirpee" type) should be worn by the radiation safety officer at all times while he is investigating a radiation incident. Several companies are now manufacturing and distributing these instruments.

B) The radiation safety officer should wear a film badge to record any exposure which he may receive during his investigation of an incident.

C) It is necessary to have available and operational a portable instrument for sampling the air in which the radium bank or sources have been located. This is especially important when sources have been isolated in a closed closet for a long period of time.

D) An alpha-beta-gamma ray survey meter with a thin end window Geiger-Mueller tube is necessary.

E) An accurate ion chamber of the "Juno" or "Cutie Pie" type is necessary for approximate measurements of the intensity of the various sources being investigated.

F) A small ultrasonic cleaner is a valuable device for cleaning and decontaminating the handling tools in a radium bank.

G) A good commercial cleansing agent such as Versene, Turco, or other similar detergent is needed for cleanup following a radium accident.

H) Various supplies such as gloves, coveralls, rags, caps, glasses, etc., as listed by Saenger (1) and Braestrup, and in *Handbook #73* (3), are necessary.

I) If the radiation hazard is due to ambient radon, it will be necessary for the radiation safety officer to wear an air pack upon his back in order to reduce the amount of radon which he inhales to tolerable levels.

When a radium accident occurs, the equipment and supplies needed should be available as a kit which can be carried quickly to any spot where the consultant or health physicist is needed. When he arrives, a complete history of the particular incident should be taken. Information as to the intensity of the sources involved, the general description of the area, the personnel involved, and what actually happened when the suspected source was broken if this is known, must be obtained. When the history has been taken, the radiation physicist should have all of his equipment and protective clothing in readiness. His monitor should be turned on, and his equipment put in an area outside the facilities whose contamination is suspected. If the leaking source is known, it should be removed, in a shielded container which has been placed inside a plastic bag, to some point perhaps 100 to 200 feet from the room in which the physicist is working. The remaining sources, even if they are not leaking, should also be removed in shielded containers to a distant point. If it is not known for certain whether any of the other sources are leaking, leak tests must be performed on them to make sure that no additional problems will arise after the area has been decontaminated.

Following removal of the radiation sources from the room in which they were stored, a complete gamma radiation survey should be done with a scintillation counter, and a yellow chalk marker used to indicate all sites of contamination. Next, an alpha-particle proportional counter or alpha-particle Geiger-Mueller counter survey should be done and areas of contamination marked. It will then be possible by using gamma-ray and alpha-particle survey meters to separate the clean or uncontaminated utensils from the contaminated utensils and place them into two separate trays. The contaminated tools can then be decontaminated with the ultrasonic cleaner or with the detergents. At the same time, the sink can be used, if it is not contaminated, to clean porous materials and to soak and further clean other items.

All items which cannot be decontaminated, and those which are of such value that further effort will make them more costly than their original or replacement value, should be discarded. Paper or plastic bags which can be disposed of to an authorized radioactive waste collector can be used to collect contaminated items. These should not be returned to the room where the radium sources are held. The sources should be thoroughly washed before they are put back into any of the clean storage areas, since it is quite likely that they have collected radon daughter products over an extended period of time.

After the area has been decontaminated to a satisfactory level, it will be permissible to return the radium sources to their storage place. A radiation survey is then conducted with an accurate ion chamber device, and a report submitted to the person responsible for the radium storage area. This report should include residual contamination levels, the results of the radiation survey, and any recommendations for follow-up tests and surveys which need to be conducted at the facility.

The leaking sources should be returned to the manufacturers for reencapsulation. If this is not worthwhile, they can be disposed of in the radioactive "garbage." The suggested actions given above are only a very general outline of the steps which can be taken in handling radiation incidents or radium accidents of a very low level.

If the area in which action is to be taken, such as that which may be found in a contaminated radium bank, is highly contaminated, most of the steps to be taken will be the same. It probably will be necessary to use a portable air pack similar to a diver's oxygen supply system. It will also be necessary to monitor the air thoroughly before one enters the room in which the radium accident took place. In addition, personnel should use disposable clothing rather than the cotton coveralls which may be used in a low-level radium accident. Here, it is quite likely that such clothing will have to be discarded following the cleanup.

REFERENCES

1. Saenger, E. L., ed.: *Medical Aspects of Radiation Accidents.* U.S. Government Printing Office, Washington, D.C., 1963.
2. NBS Handbook 69, *Maximum Permissible Body Burdens and Maximum Permissible Concentrations of Radionuclides in Air and in Water for Occupational Exposure.* Recommendations of the NCRP, U.S. Government Printing Office, Washington, D.C., 1959.
3. Hale, John: A Method for Testing Radium Containers for Leaking Using the Well-type Scintillation Counter. *Radiology, 72*:105, January 1959.
4. NBS Handbook 73, *Protection Against Radiations from Sealed Gamma Sources.* Recommendations of the NCRP, Report No. 24; U.S. Government Printing Office, Washington, D.C., 1960.

DISCUSSION

Mr. G. F. Meyers (Illinois State Department of Public Health): Mr. Fields, which of the various methods for leak testing of radium do you feel is the most accurate; and would you compare it to other methods?

Mr. T. Fields: Of the methods which we have tested ourselves, we feel that the greatest accuracy is obtained by choosing a test which will combine both the leak and wipe test methods. The only one which, I believe, will give a value that I can accept and that has proven to be reproducible is the Hale test. This is the test in which activated charcoal is used. We add a refinement in our modification of the method by using various cleansing agents. We believe that we remove any removable contamination that was present on the radium needles.

There is an important consideration here. As I mentioned earlier, lead-210 actually emits a gamma ray. Therefore, whenever you do a leak and wipe test and you find that the needle is not radioactively clean, you can identify lead-210 contamination. In my experience, I have never found a clean radium source. What I do then is to ascribe a certain amount of non-removable contamination to the radium needle. The only way you can do this is with the Hale test.

Dr. A. F. Phillips (Hurley Hospital, Flint, Michigan): Could Mr. Fields tell us at what age the pressure of helium requires resealing a radium source?

Mr. T. Fields: I don't have an answer for that. There are regulations in various states, I know, that require one to have his sources resealed at the end of ten years. This might be a good number. There are some testing techniques available which would allow us to measure the pressure in the radium needles. I think, right now, though, the practice is that, if a source is ten years old, it should be resealed. I will go along with that practice because, in all ten-year-old sources, I have found a significant amount of leakage.

Chairman W. B. Rivkin (Health Physics Associates, Highland Park, Illinois): I think there is a gentleman in the audience who can comment on this question. Would you care to comment, Dr. Landauer?

Dr. R. S. Landauer: I believe that a value which has been reported is that, for an average 10-milligram radium needle, twenty-five years old, there is an estimated pressure of a few ounces per square millimeter. In the paper, as I recall, the authors gave their values in pounds per square foot. If you reduce this to volumes in which you are interested, it comes to just a couple of ounces per square millimeter, which is not very much.

Another problem, though, is not the formation of helium in the radium needle, but the dissociation of water that may have been in the radium when it was sealed. I believe that this is a much more significant matter. If the radium was dry when it was sealed, there is comparatively little chance of pressure building up.

I would like to make one comment about Mr. Fields's Hale test. I believe that it is entirely too sensitive. It will detect radon leakages of the order of magnitude of simple diffusion of radon through the platinum walls of the needle. The result is, as Mr. Fields said, that practically every radium needle that is tested by this method shows a leakage. I believe that we should use a less sensitive test, such as the ordinary cotton test.

Mr. T. Fields: I agree with Dr. Landauer that the Hale test is very sensitive. The problem encountered with other tests is that you can't really get a repeatable value or say, "Yes, I can do this test and get the same numbers out of it the next time I do the test." When you use the Hale test—and it is relatively simple—you do get repeatability and sensitivity. We don't require a lot of sensitivity, and right now we use the value of less than 0.005 microcuries of removable radon in twenty-four hours to detect a leaking source. If the value is less than that, we accept the source as satisfactory.

It is questionable whether 0.005 microcuries in twenty-four hours is significant. I know there have been suggestions that it is a hazard level. When you are out in practice and have to accept responsibility for your decisions, it is good to have such a value to use.

RADIATION MONITORING AND NON-NUCLEAR WEAPONS ACCIDENTS

WILLIAM S. JOHNSON, SR.

Eberline Instrument Corporation
Santa Fe, New Mexico

THE SCATTERING of large quantities of plutonium-239 over sizeable land areas is a situation unique to the non-nuclear detonation of nuclear weapons. Fortunately, such accidents are not a common occurrence. They have been investigated most thoroughly as a part of specific field operations involving deliberate detonations.

The most extensive field operation to date was Operation ROLLER COASTER conducted in the spring of 1963 at the Tonopah Test Range, Nevada. ROLLER COASTER was the joint effort of the U.S. Atomic Energy Commission, the Department of Defense, and the United Kingdom, and included four detonations. This paper is a report on one of the projects which was a part of the total field operation, namely, Project 2.5—Alpha Survey, which the Eberline Instrument Corporation was selected to perform.

Project Objectives

The assigned objectives of Project 2.5 were:

a) To provide a large-area radiac* survey of the plutonium-contaminated areas and to establish contamination level contours.

b) To correlate, by chemical analysis, radiac meter readings of plutonium contamination with absolute surface levels of plutonium deposition.

c) To investigate the feasibility of portable and mobile low-energy electromagnetic radiation detection techniques for plutonium contamination over extended land surfaces.

For the purposes of this paper, only objectives (a) and (c) are

*Radiac is a term used frequently in U.S. Department of Defense publications. It refers to radiation measurements in health physics and is derived from the underlined letters of these words: radiation detection, indication and computation.

considered. Radiochemical analysis of soil samples for deposited plutonium content has not been completed at this time and is not ready to be reported on. Only meager correlative data between radiac and radiochemistry are available. This fact precludes any conclusive statements for the present.

Operations

Each of the four detonations was carried out under different placement conditions. These were as follows:

Shot No. 1. Open, i.e., no cover, on steel plate mounted on reinforced concrete slab; approximately 100 pounds of explosive yield.

Shot No. 2. Open, i.e., no cover, on reinforced concrete slab; approximately 900 pounds of explosive yield.

Shot No. 3. In stored configuration with two feet of earth overburden; approximately 2000 pounds of explosive yield.

Shot No. 4. In stored configuration with eight feet of earth overburden; approximately 2000 pounds of explosive yield.

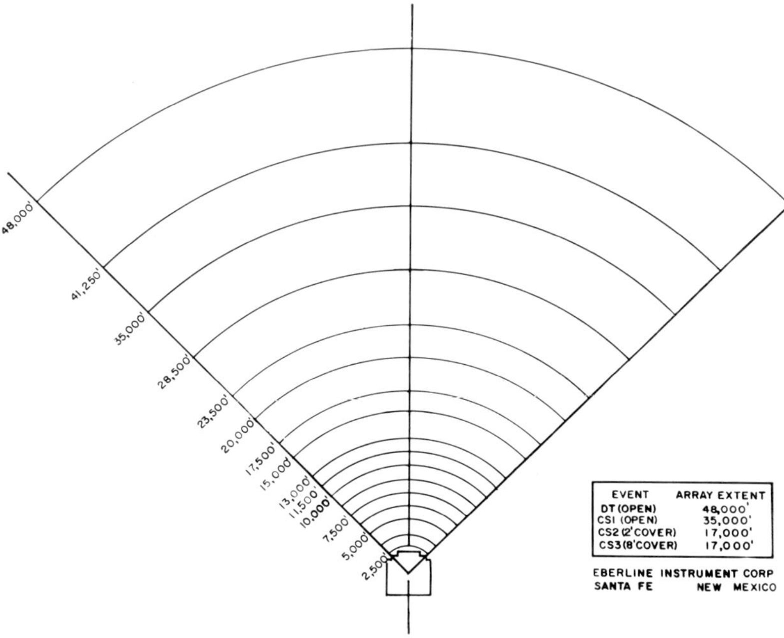

FIGURE V-1. Downwind array of instrumented arcs.

The plutonium-239 available for dissemination in each shot was essentially constant.

The array of downwind alpha-particle monitoring stations was similar for each event, differing only in the distance downwind to which they extended (Figure V-1). Each of the four arrays covered a section of the test range not previously contaminated by prior weapons tests at the Nevada Test Site, or by a prior shot of ROLLER COASTER. Shot No. 1 had the most extensive station array—out to 48,000 feet; Shot No. 2—35,000 feet; Shots 3 and 4—17,500 feet.

A 90° sector was selected for instrumentation; meteorological restrictions were such as to place the downwind fallout within this sector. This was accomplished successfully for each shot. Alpha monitoring stations were located every ¾ degree on arcs across the 90° sector (121 stations per arc). A crude road was cut along each arc to facilitate movement of vehicles over the desert terrain. Each station consisted of a 12″ x 12″ x 1″ brushed concrete pad as the alpha-particle monitoring surface. A previous field operation in 1957 had

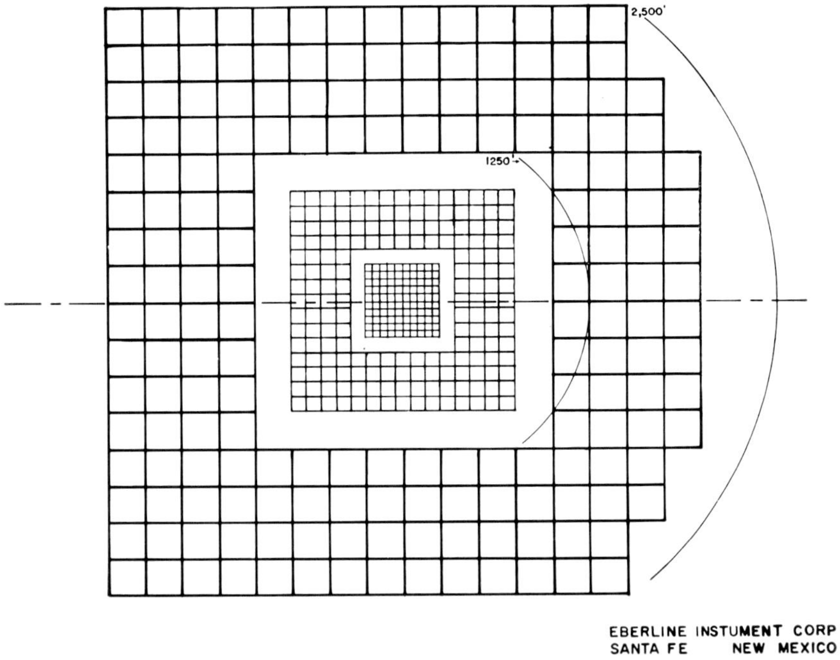

FIGURE V-2. Close-in array of instrumented locations.

established the validity of measuring alpha-particle emitter contamination levels on a common surface, and suitability of a surface consisting of a brushed concrete pad.

Since most shots were detonated during the early morning hours, it was necessary for alpha-particle monitoring to be delayed until daylight. At this time, ten two-man monitoring teams in three-quarter ton weapons carriers equipped with two-way radios were dispatched to assigned arcs. Information obtained from mobile low-energy gamma-ray detectors, to be described later, was used to select that portion of each arc which was likely to yield positive contamination data. Monitoring continued at each station across the arc until an area with 100 cpm/probe or less was reached. Periodic reports were transmitted via radio to permit plots of current contamination levels to be maintained at a central location. A team was then assigned a second arc, if necessary to complete the survey. Four to five hours were required for this operation.

Concurrently, a similar survey was being performed in the immediate vicinity of the detonation point by additional monitoring teams. Here, a rectangular pattern of brushed concrete pads (from 50 to 250 feet apart) was used (Figure V-2). This survey usually took an hour longer than arc surveys, as team members performed additional duties such as a reconnaissance of the zero point and of the debris scattered by the detonation.

Re-surveys for early weathering effects were planned but, in one of the anomalies of the desert, 1963 was a wet spring, and these could be accomplished only after the first shot. Subsequent shots were followed by rain in the period from nine to twenty-four hours following the shot, which meant more "weathering" than had been expected.

Instrumentation and Calibration

The basic instrument for determining surface alpha-particle emitter contamination was the Eberline Instrument Corporation Model PAC-3G Portable Gas Proportional Alpha Counter (Figure V-3). This instrument was selected because of its ability to provide reliable and reproducible information in the environment of the Tonopah Test Range.

The Model PAC-3G has a detecting probe with approximately

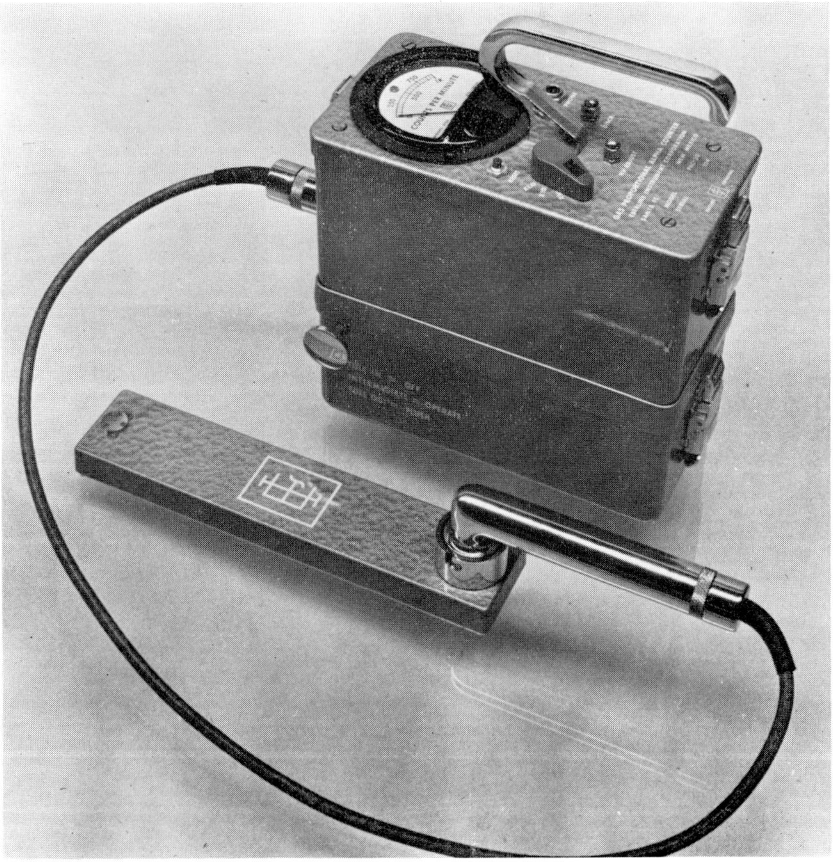

FIGURE V-3. Portable Gas Proportional Alpha Particle Counter, Model PAC-3G.

60 cm^2 of sensitive area. Its window is 0.85 mg/cm^2. The rate meter readout operates over three ranges: 0-1,000 cpm, 0-10,000 cpm, and 0-100,000 cpm. A "times 20" shield is available to extend the range to 2×10^6 cpm if necessary.

The procedure was to monitor each concrete pad in three locations by placing the "feet" of the probe in contact. A set of calibrated plutonium-239 standards was provided to each field team. Instrument calibration was checked and recorded after reading each concrete pad on the range in which the pad measurements fell. These field sources were 1⅛ inch diameter discs and served as secondary standards. Primary calibration was against plutonium-239 extended-area sources.

Instruments were calibrated to read 100 per cent of the 2π emission rate of these sources. Figure V-4 shows both the disc and extended-area sources.

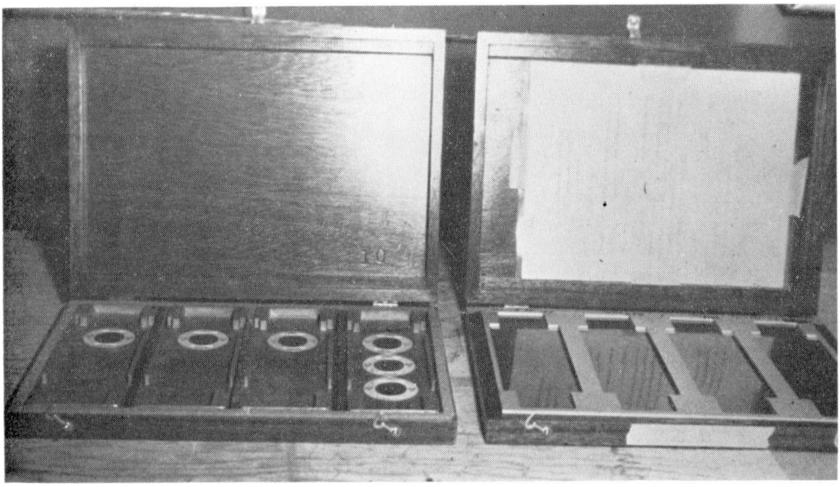

FIGURE V-4. Discs (*left*) and extended area (*right*) alpha-particle calibration sources.

It should be recalled that one of the objectives of Project 2.5 was a feasibility study of portable and mobile low-energy gamma-ray detectors. Strictly speaking, the plutonium-239 photon radiations are approximately 17-kev x-rays; however, in the consideration of the overall electromagnetic spectrum available for detection, common usage refers to them as "low-energy gamma-rays."

The portable probe was the Eberline Model PG-1 Plutonium Gamma Probe which utilizes the Eberline Model PAC-ISA electronics (Figure V-5). This probe has a photomultiplier tube, crystal, and window encased in a ruggedized housing. The crystal is 1 mm thick sodium iodide, thallium activated [NaI(T1)], covered with a 1 mil aluminum window. This combination of probe and electronics is used in the field with the probe held approximately 30 inches above the surface. In this manner, the detector is "seeing" a circular area approaching six feet in diameter. In the absence of a uniformly distributed plutonium source of this size, the PG-1 meter was calibrated only provisionally. This was done using 1⅛ inch disc sources with

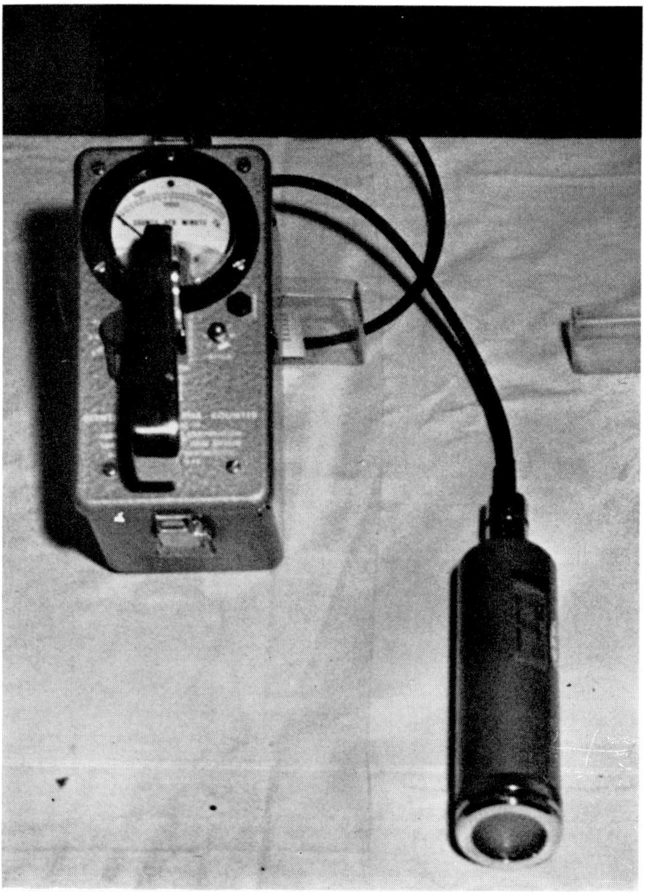

FIGURE V-5. Portable Plutonium Gamma Ray Probe, Model PG-1, with Electronics and Readout Case, Model PAC-ISA.

activity levels up to 2×10^7 dpm plutonium-239. The probe was placed in contact with these sources and set to read 3 per cent of the 2π alpha emission rate.

Background (natural activity plus circuit noise) is an important consideration in setting up this instrument. Arbitrarily, the DISC setting was selected to give 2,000 to 3,000 cpm "background." It is to be emphasized that the PG-1 probe is of value as a detector rather than as an absolute measuring device. It was designed with this limitation in mind, and applications beyond this would require special conditions of calibration and of contamination deposition.

The mobile low-energy gamma-ray detector involved the installation of detector and electronics on and in a conventional panel truck (Figure V-6). The detector is a two and one-half inch diameter by one inch thick NaI (Tl) crystal with a 1 mil aluminum window mounted on a three inch photomultiplier tube. This was housed inside a two inch thick lead shield mounted on the front of the vehicle, with a crystal thirty inches from the ground.

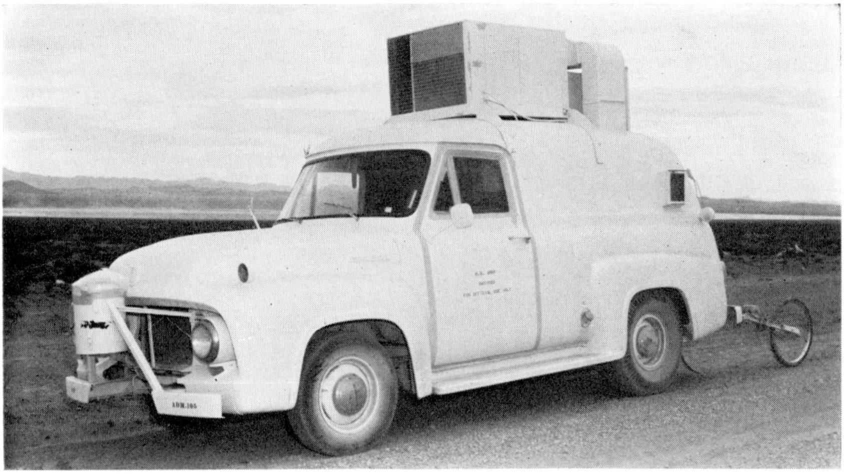

FIGURE V-6. External view of mobile low energy gamma-ray unit.

The electronics were located inside the vehicle, facing forward on the right side (Figure V-7). They consisted of two single-channel pulse height analyzers (Radiation Instrument Development Laboratory, Inc.) and associated amplifier, power supplies and cabinet. The duplex recorder (Minneapolis-Honeywell) with selsyn paper drive was mounted on this cabinet.

A motor-generator set was mounted in the rear of the vehicle and separated from the operator's section by a sealed plywood partition (Figure V-8). A 24,000 BTU/hr refrigerated air conditioner (York) was mounted on top of the vehicle. The drive mechanism for the recorder selsyn paper drive consisted of a twenty-four inch bicycle wheel and two chain-driven sprockets. This yielded paper speeds from 40 yd/in to 200 yd/in. The exterior of the panel truck was painted white for maximum heat reflection. All cracks and holes were sealed to make the interior as free of dust as possible.

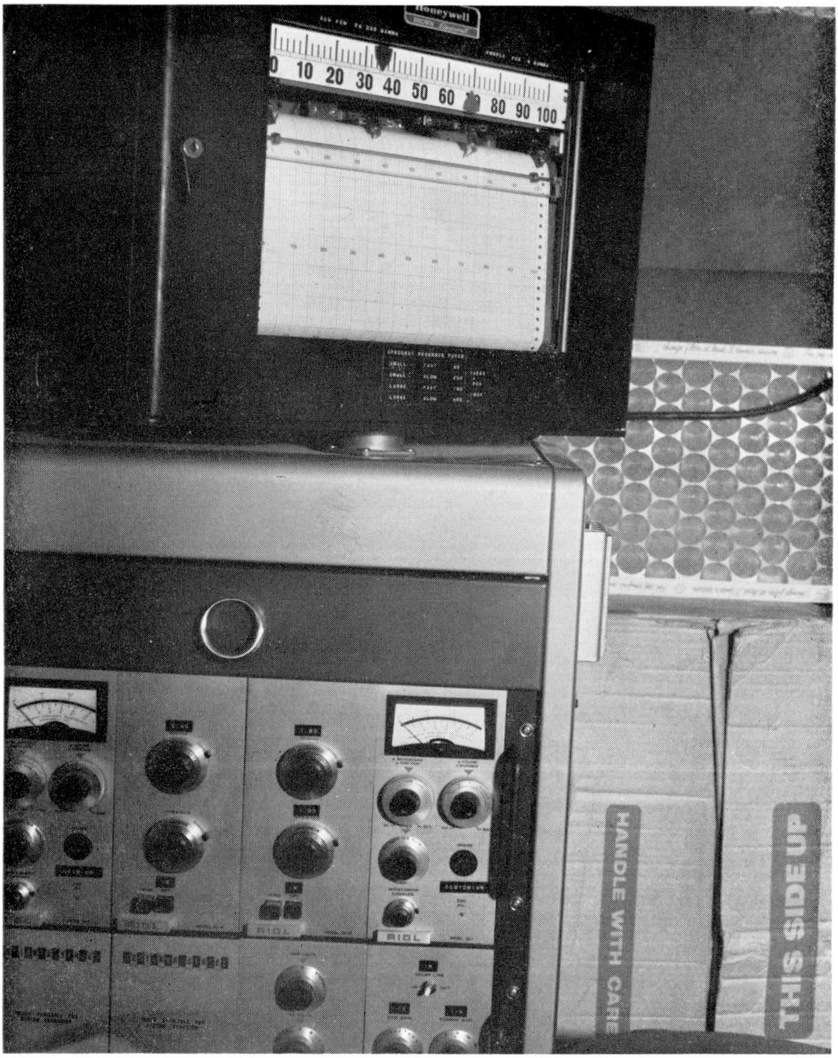

FIGURE V-7. Internal view of mobile low energy gamma-ray unit showing dual pen recorder and electronics cabinet.

Two channels of spectral analysis were provided so as to permit the detection of any other gamma-ray energies simultaneously with the 17-kev photons from plutonium-239. Calibration was performed with a one and one-eighth inch disc standard held in contact with the crystal window. A typical pulse spectrum from such a calibration is

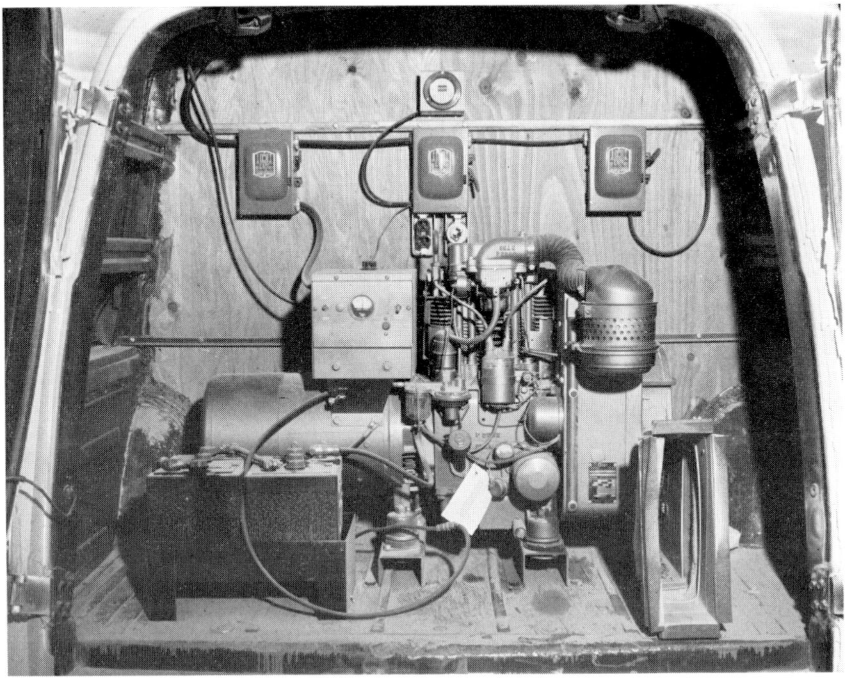

FIGURE V-8. View of mobile low energy gamma-ray unit inside rear doors.

shown in Figure V-9. Based on this information and its substantiation by field measurements of surface deposition, the channels were set on the 17- and 60-kev peaks.

The same electronics and detector were duplicated, though not mounted on a vehicle, for purposes of assaying large quantities of soil overburden for its scavenging effect (Figure V-10). This operation was not a part of the Alpha Survey Project, but is reported on here as another application of this detection technique. The soil entered a moving belt from a hopper-shaker-hopper arrangement, and was laid down at a depth of approximately two inches. Several hundred cubic yards were assayed for plutonium-239 by this method.

Results

At this time, all results must be considered as semi-quantitative at best. An extensive radiochemical program is currently in progress to provide absolute determination of plutonium-239 deposition. These

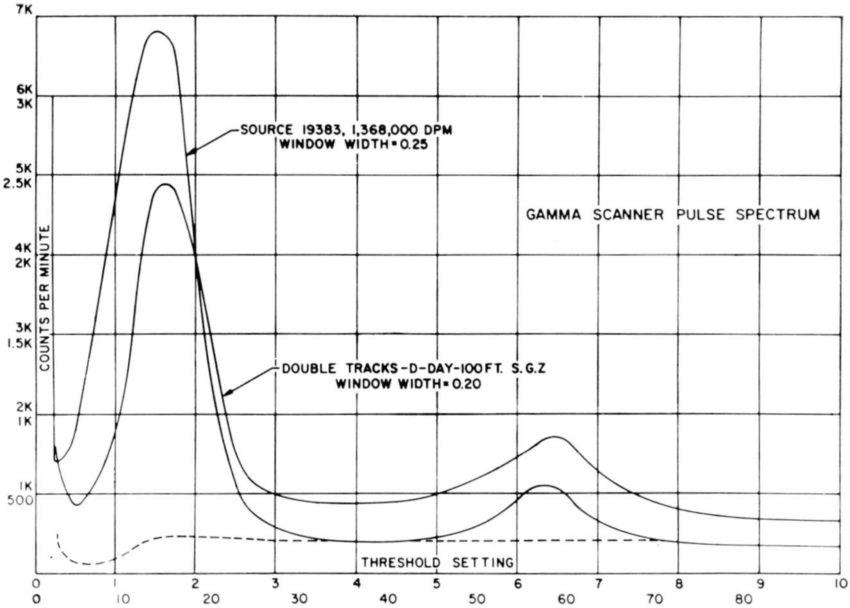

FIGURE V-9. Gamma-ray spectrum of standard plutonium source and post-detonation debris.

data will be correlated with field alpha-particle and gamma-ray measurements to yield appropriate conversion factors.

The preliminary downwind contamination contours are presented in Figures V-11, V-12, V-13 and V-14. Patterns vary from extremely narrow limits to one which covers practically the entire instrumented array. Superimposed on Figure V-15 is the contamination pattern as developed from mobile low-energy gamma-ray detectors. While these detectors are not quite as sensitive as those giving straight alpha-particle measurements, they can operate in situations which are not optimum for alpha-particle detection, e.g., in inclement weather, heavy vegetation, and forested areas. Also, considering the comfort and safety of personnel and the speed and thoroughness of data collection, this method may actually be superior where rapid delineation of contamination patterns over large land areas is desirable. As noted in Figure V-16, the solid dark line shows the peak surface concentration to lie between the grid intersections. Also, one-tenth of the peak lies nearly between these same intersections. Without the continuous trace

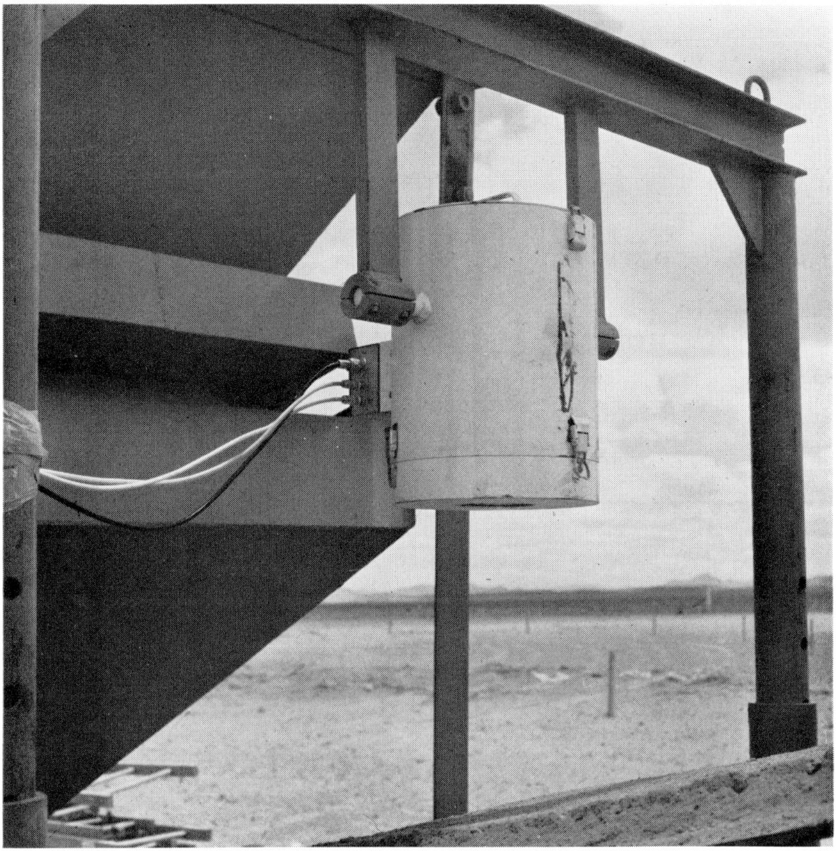

FIGURE V-10. Soil Assay Unit. Detector, shield and preamplifier (*center*); hopper and shaker (*left*); belt carrying soil for assay (*bottom*).

of the mobile detectors, about 90 per cent of this information could be missed by portable alpha-particle monitoring devices even with this high density of stations.

Certainly, brushed concrete surfaces proved to be a reliable method for obtaining a preliminary assessment of contamination levels. A practical result is the fact that relatively flat surfaces of nearly any composition should be used as the monitored medium whenever they are available. Portable alpha-particle detectors, supplemented by portable low-energy gamma-ray detectors, serve adequately as the basic instruments for immediate response to weapon accidents in-

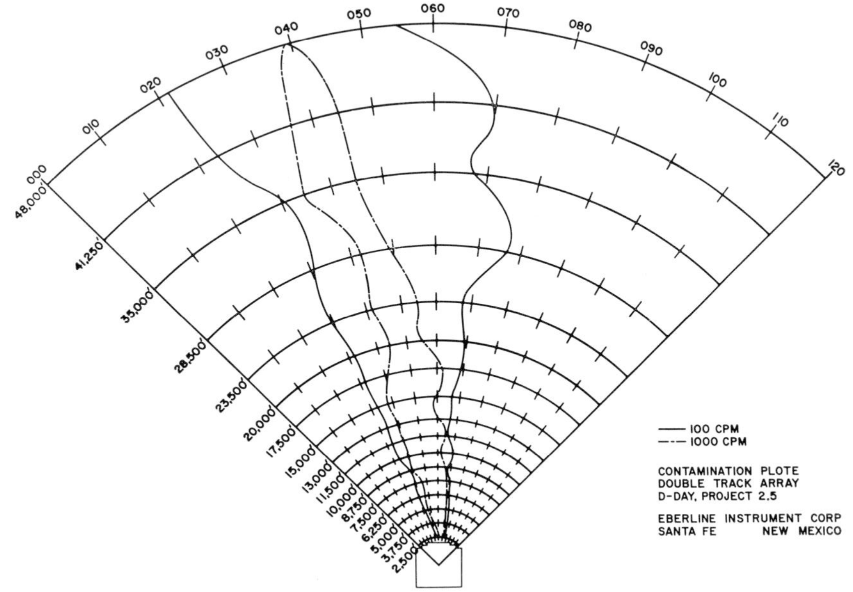

FIGURE V-11. Contamination plot, cpm, with PAC-3G probe. Double tracks event–Operation ROLLER COASTER.

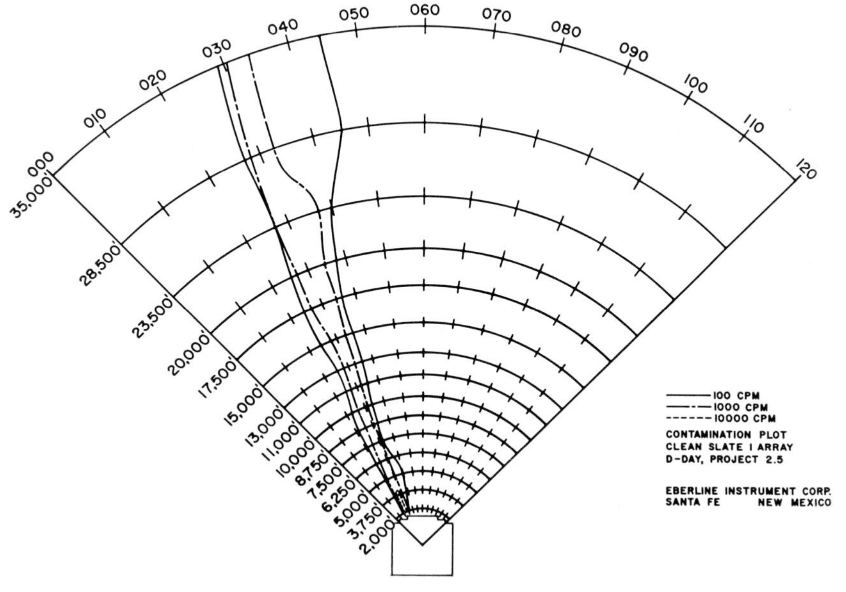

FIGURE V-12. Contamination plot, cpm, with PAC-3G probe. Clean slate-one event–Operation ROLLER COASTER.

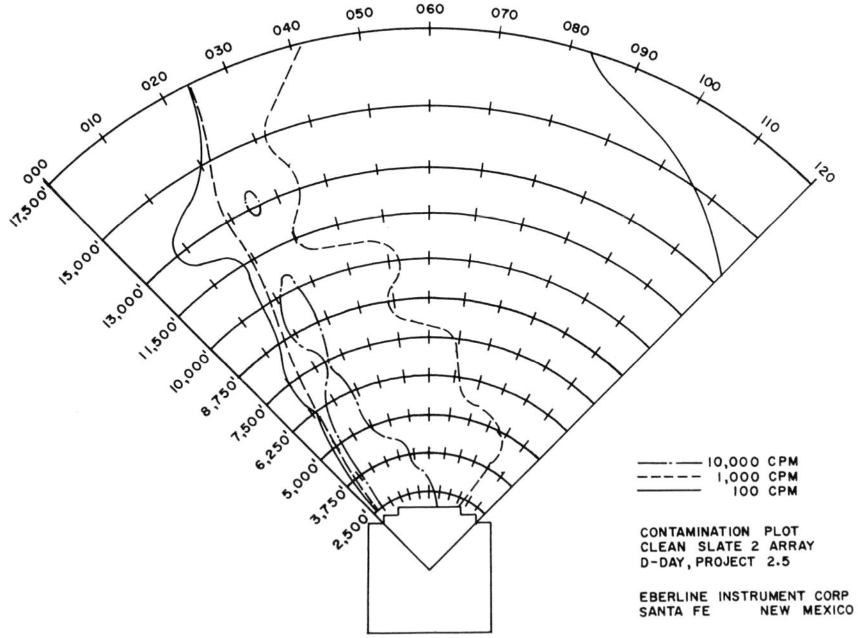

FIGURE V-13. Contamination plot, cpm, with PAC-3G probe. Clean slate-two event–Operation ROLLER COASTER.

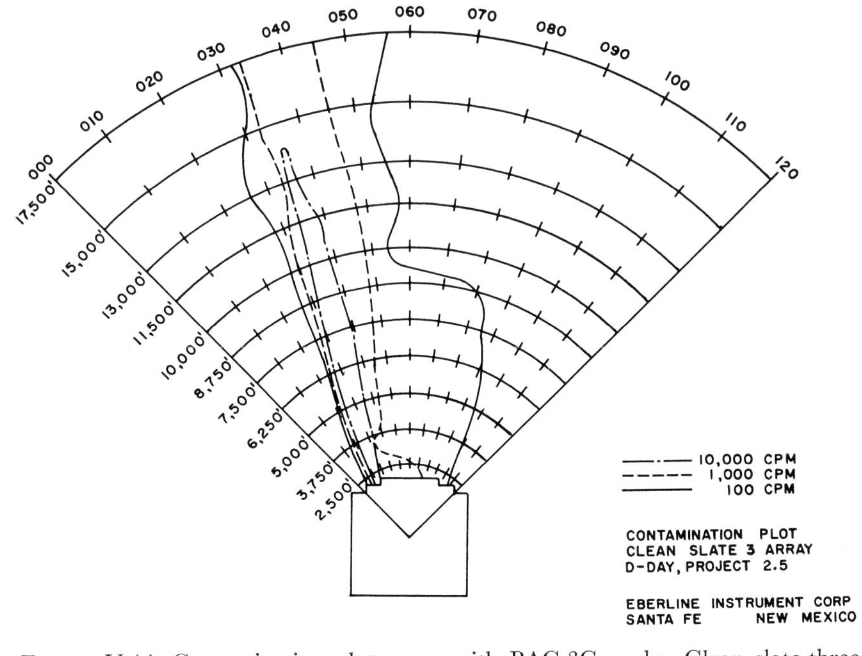

FIGURE V-14. Contamination plot, cpm, with PAC-3G probe. Clean slate-three event–Operation ROLLER COASTER.

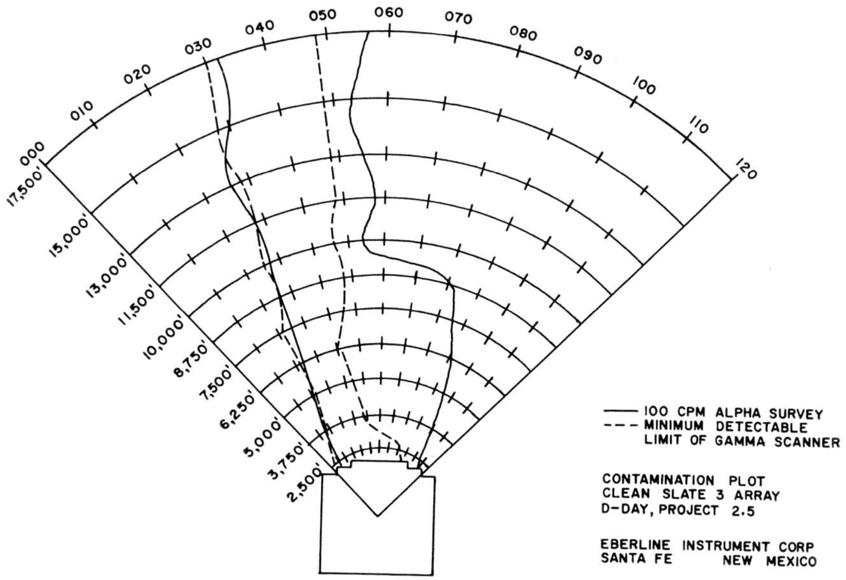

FIGURE V-15. Contamination plot—portable instrument and mobile low energy gamma-ray unit. Clean slate-three event—Operation ROLLER COASTER (compare with Figure V-14).

volving a non-nuclear detonation. A word of caution is necessary, however, namely, to include an initial gamma-ray survey in emergency planning against the occurrence of a small fission contribution which can create hazardous levels of external whole-body radiation. The presence or absence of this radiation must be established as the first step in the radiological survey.

In regard to other radiological safety practices, Operation ROLLER COASTER was conducted without any particularly restrictive personal protective requirements. Anti-contamination clothing such as coveralls, shoe covers, caps and gloves was used in all areas. Valid air sampling information is difficult if not impossible to obtain in work areas of a field operation. For this reason, respiratory protective equipment should always be worn when the preliminary assessment of the contamination pattern is being developed. In ROLLER COASTER the U.S. Army Model M-17 Full Face Mask was used exclusively with excellent results, not only in regard to the pro-

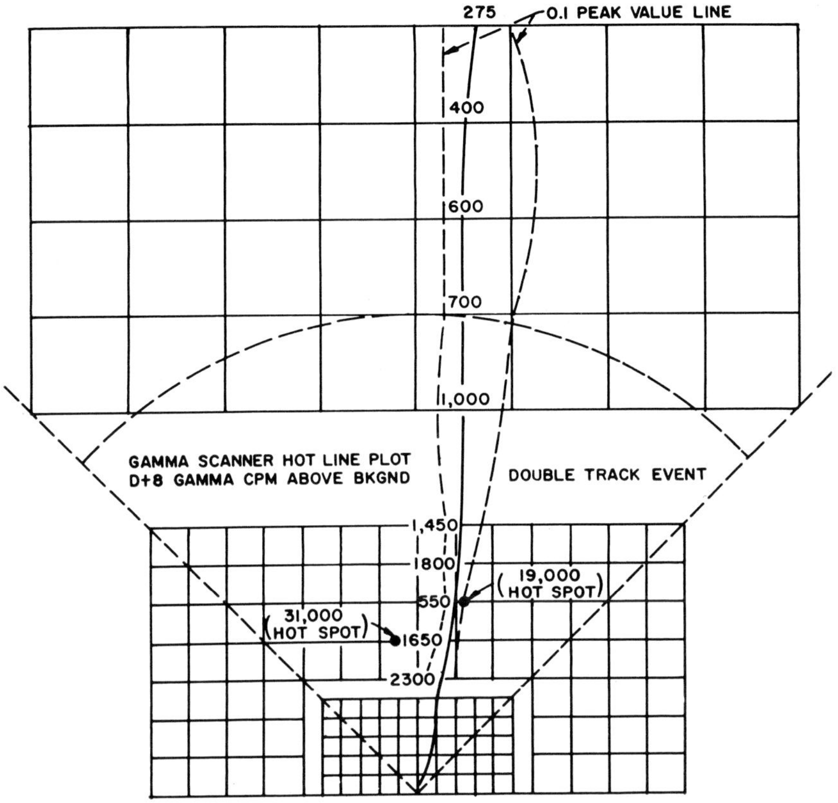

FIGURE V-16. D + 8 day mobile low energy gamma-ray plot of close-in deposition. Double tracks event—Operation ROLLER COASTER.

tection provided, but also in operator comfort. It was found to be adequate in all work areas.

Conclusion

The experience gained in Operation ROLLER COASTER offers additional insight into the radiological problems associated with nuclear weapon accidents. These experiences are being evaluated at this time and will be reported on completely in documents to be published in the near future. For the present, however, it can be stated that the means are available to assess the contamination problem adequately and safely. In view of the valuable contributions made by low-energy gamma-ray detectors, it can be forecast with confidence that the technique of using these detectors will find further applications as a useful tool in emergency situations.

DOSIMETRY AND INSTRUMENTS FOR ACCIDENT SITUATION ASSESSMENT

HOWARD R. FISH, JR.
Argonne National Laboratory
Argonne, Illinois

ANYONE WHO HAS never experienced a serious radioactive "spill" or an accident involving high radiation levels may tend to underestimate the consequences. Proper handling of such a situation demands that information be readily available concerning the exact location and magnitude of the radiation hazard. This is usually possible only if the instruments needed for radiation measurements are held in reserve, so that they may not be seriously involved in the accident themselves.

Equally important is good knowledge of the dose accumulated by personnel involved, both at the time of occurrence and during the exercise of control and decontamination procedures. Combined knowledge of these factors will enable the person or persons responsible for health physics to work with the confidence and efficiency approaching that of the properly equipped firefighter.

Some guides are presented here to assist those responsible persons whose primary occupation is not that of a health physicist. Many of the necessary items are briefly described, together with their proper applications. Problems connected with maintaining them in a condition of readiness may be relieved by the procedures recommended here.

Instruments

A. ***Dose-integrating Instruments (Dosimeters).*** Personnel dosimeters are those commonly used to measure the dose of ionizing radiation received by an individual during a given period of exposure. All of the various types are sufficiently small and light in weight to be easily worn on the person.

The pocket dosimeter is one traditional type. It consists of a quartz fiber electroscope coupled to an ion chamber. The unit is readied for use by applying an electrical charge of about 150 volts, so that the indicating fiber is repelled to zero on the scale. As the chamber intercepts radiation, it discharges and measures the ionization produced by the penetrating (gamma-rays, hard beta particles, or neutrons) radiation. Logically, the auxiliary device used to apply the required charge is called a "charger." This charger is usually battery powered and usually compatible only with a specific type of quartz fiber dosimeter.

The advantages of the quartz fiber dosimeter are:

1) It yields fairly accurate information quickly and is reasonably uniform in its response to radiations in the energy range of 50 kev to 2 mev.

2) It is economical for long-term use and may be recharged with simple and inexpensive chargers.

3) It is reliable and requires little maintenance.

The disadvantages of the quartz fiber dosimeter are:

1) There is no permanent record.

2) Frequent reading, tabulating, and recharging may be required.

3) It will not withstand severe shock.

4) Its range of measurement is limited; however, full-scale ranges of 10, 20, and 100 roentgens are available.

A newer type of ion chamber dosimeter features an audible alarm when an exposure reaches a specified dose. Models are available designed to sound an alarm when a dose of 1, 5, or 25 R is received. If these are used at dose rates higher than those that will cause an alarm in one minute, inaccuracy results which will become greater as the dose rate increases. Such an instrument weighs approximately one pound, has good battery life and a uniform response to gamma-ray energies from 50 kev to 1.5 mev.

The film badge is another widely used type of personnel dosimeter. It usually consists of a plastic holder containing dental-size photographic film packets, and is worn on the person as a continuous monitor of particulate or gamma radiation. After exposure, the film is processed, read on a densitometer, and interpreted. By means of simultaneous use of various emulsions, a wide range of dosages can be measured. For low dosages of neutrons (up to 10 rem and with no more than 1 rad of electromagnetic radiation), a special film with a tracking emulsion is employed. The use of cadmium and other metal filters over portions of the film enables definition of the energy range to which the films have been exposed, by comparison of the densities of these portions of the processed film.

The advantages of the various film badges are:

1) They are reliable, since there is good uniformity within batches of emulsion.

2) They have a wide range of dose response, from 25 mR to 3,000 R; by special processing this can be extended to 10,000 R.

3) They provide a permanent record of the period of use.

The disadvantages of film badges are:

1) They require careful processing, densitometer reading, and interpretation to determine the results.

2) They require storage in locations where extraneous exposures will not accumulate.

3) They must be changed periodically to insure uniform results.

Fixed-location dosimeters may also be used to good advantage if placed in areas where there is a high probability of severe exposures. Some of the various types which might be used are:

1) Film packets containing several high-range films.

2) Thermoluminescent powder dosimeters.

3) Integrating ion-chamber instruments with alarms.

4) Various activation types for neutrons.

B. ***Rate-measuring Instruments (Dose or Disintegration Rate).*** Instruments for the detection and measurement of radioactivity and the measurement of dose rates from penetrating radiations fall into the general categories of hand-carried portable (survey meters) and the larger, fixed or mobile, ones. Which of many possible choices should be available for accident assessment will, of course, depend on the nature of the hazards. The various means of detection should be considered first; therefore, comments on the radiation detector component of these instruments are in order. Examples (by names or descriptions) of situations in which these detectors are employed will be given.

ALPHA-PARTICLE DETECTORS. Detectors for *alpha-particle emitters* and their associated instruments are:

1) The older air proportional counters which use various thin window materials exhibit rather unstable characteristics, especially in humid environments. They have been employed in portable survey meters and personnel monitors in a wide variety of shapes and sizes (often with nylon windows of 0.05 to 0.10 mil thickness).

2) Gas proportional counters have now largely replaced the air proportional detectors in portable instruments. They use 0.25 mil aluminized Mylar windows (with a sensitive area of 60 - 100 cm^2) which greatly improve their stability and resistance to mechanical damage. The counting gas commonly used is a 99 per cent pure grade of propane which may present an explosion hazard. The gas is metered very slowly into the sensitive volume of the counter, so that a slight positive pressure (with respect to atmospheric) is maintained.

3) Large sensitive area gas proportional counters (of 250 to 300 cm^2) are used in personnel or floor monitors. The usual counting gas is either the 99 per cent propane or a 90 per cent argon—10 per cent methane mixture known as "P-10." Although P-10 is non-flammable, it is not condensable and, therefore, must be stored in large, heavy steel cylinders. This is a distinct disadvantage when it is used in portable or mobile instruments.

4) Alpha-particle scintillation detectors, like the gas proportional detectors, have a thin window which must be kept light-tight. Sensitive areas of 100 cm^2 are common in the portable types, and units as large as 200 cm^2 are used in personnel monitors.

5) For highly contaminated areas, thin-windowed ion chamber detectors are best. Among the instruments using this detector are the Samson, Juno, and the newer low-energy survey meters.

6) Where great sensitivity is required, the 2π internal gas-flow proportional counters are used either without windows or with extremely thin ones. A sample (such as a smear) must be placed into the counter.

BETA-RAY DETECTORS. *Beta radiation emitter* detectors and the instruments in which they find application are:

1) Geiger-Mueller (GM) tubes with 30 mg/cm^2 windows are sensitive to intermediate-energy beta-particles and low-energy gamma radiations. They are widely used in survey meters as well as in the larger mobile and fixed instruments, because they are rugged, dependable, and require relatively simple circuitry.

legal use of such documents, before they are filed away following the radiation accident.

E. Eye Witness Accounts

Eye witness accounts of a radiation accident provide essential documentation that can be extremely valuable, especially if they are obtained shortly after the incident when facts are fresh in the person's mind. One of the best times to obtain such information is immediately after the required health physics and medical procedures have been completed and the individual has had a chance to regain his composure. Written statements should be obtained from any individual potentially exposed as a result of the radiation accident, or who claims to have been affected by it, as well as from those persons who may have pertinent information concerning the accident. These statements can be in the form of tape recordings or of hand-written narrative reports of what the individual saw, did, and saw others doing; also, where and when certain events relative to the accident took place. Such an individual should also describe how and why he believes the accident occurred. These accounts should not be prepared as a cooperative or "team effort," nor should they be written under the "helpful eye" of a supervisor. They need not be in scholarly prose, but should be clear and accurate accounts in the individual's own words. Each should be signed and dated by the individual. Again, a tape recording of this report which is later typed, signed by the individual and dated may be used. It is recommended that reports of this type be witnessed or notarized.

When such statements are reviewed by an experienced investigator, they sometimes produce clues which may be extremely important in reconstructing pertinent facts at the time of the accident and determining its cause and practical methods of avoiding recurrences. Such statements have uncovered other undetected or unreported accidents that had occurred in the past. For example, in investigating the statement made by a radiographer during one radiographic accident, we learned about two others involving the same piece of equipment, but of lesser severity.

F. Photographic Reenactments

Photographic reenactments of the radiation accident are invaluable in establishing the location and identity of the individuals with respect to the radiation source. Eye witness accounts are used to reconstruct the scene. A non-radioactive "dummy" radioisotope source is set up to duplicate the actual conditions during the radiation accident. Either the individuals involved in the incident or substitutes are asked to attempt to duplicate as closely as possible the actions which took place. We have used at least one and sometimes several motion picture cameras as well as still cameras to photograph such reenactments.

We have found it valuable to have a narrative account of the reenactment recorded on tape. The tapes also contain periodic time checks along with announcements of the running times. That is, while the narrator describes the actions being filmed, a timekeeper can be heard in the background counting off the seconds that have elapsed during each important phase of the reenactment. Thus, when the recording is played back along with the movies, or matched with sequence photographs, determinations can be made relative to the approximate times and distances where personnel may have received significant radiation exposures. Another very valuable technique is to include in the background of the picture at least one large electric clock that has been synchronized to start at an appropriate time during the reenactment to document the running time of the various stages of the reenactment.

Documentary photographs should also be taken of the equipment present in the incident. It is our practice to use a shielded periscope to photograph a source involved in a radiation accident. In some cases, such photographs reveal wear or defects in the source or the equipment. Radiation injuries should be photographed in color and properly labeled as to date and identity of the individual. The documentary photographs together with the statements by personnel involved in the accident enable the health physicist to reconstruct the scene for the purpose of obtaining radiation dosimetry data. Polaroid photographs can be very helpful during the dosimetry experiments as well as during the reenactment.

G. Reporting of Radiation Accidents

Every organization has a policy according to which good or bad news concerning that organization is released to its own officials and to outside firms, official agencies, and eventually to the public. Unfortunately, many organizations fail to realize that they can have a radiation accident and that they may not be prepared administratively, technically, or financially to cope with such a situation. Top management may not have recognized the need for an official of the organization to become aware of the legal responsibility for reporting a radiation accident within a prescribed period of time to certain official agencies, as required by law. A responsible individual within the organization must be clearly designated and briefed as to *whom* he is to notify; *when, where,* and *how* such reports must be transmitted, and *what* should be reported.

Naturally, a radiation accident is not a type of occurrence which an organization would want anyone to know about. In fact, it may be of interest that, in our work on radiation accidents, we have detected two and possibly three cases of what psychologists refer to as "subconscious denial" on the part of radiation workers that a radiation accident had occurred. That is, an individual refused to accept the fact that he had received a potentially serious exposure.

However, top management must make clear to each radiation worker that failure to notify certain designated personnel (e.g., radiological safety officer, or a corporate official) of an accident involving radioactive materials or radiation-producing equipment can be reason for dismissal. Furthermore, all radiation workers must be made aware of their responsibilities as specified by federal regulations (1, 2) and other appropriate state and local regulations relative to their assigned duties which involve radiation safety and the preparation of radiation reports. Usually, these responsibilities are clearly defined in the operating procedures manual. Therefore, the worker involved in a radiation accident should have received prior instructions as contained in the operating procedures manual, augmented by instructions on radiation emergencies. He should know what to do to protect himself and his fellow workers in the event of an emergency, and whom to notify by using the procedure shown in Appendix VI-1. The periodic use of the check list (Appendix VI-5) will facilitate understanding and adherence to the emergency plan.

Once the notification of the radiation emergency has been received and initial action taken to get the situation under control, the magnitude of the accident must be determined in order to establish which of the various reporting procedures is to be followed as prescribed in federal regulations (1, 2, 3) as well as in appropriate state and local laws.

In order to aid key management personnel in determining the magnitude of the accident, we have prepared a table (see Appendix VI-6) for the evaluation of incidents involving radiation. The classification of the radiation accident can be established by reviewing the classification criteria and marking an "X" in the table following any statement which, at the time of the review, describes the magnitude of the situation. Depending upon the accident classification as determined by the table, appropriate notification is required in accordance with the "Radiation Incident Reporting Procedures" shown in Appendix VI-7.

It is important to note that there may be several official agencies (e.g., U.S. Atomic Energy Commission, Walsh-Healy Section of the U.S. Labor Department, state or local radiation regulatory agencies) which must be notified in accordance with their specific regulations. Figure VI-1 contains the currently available list of these agencies, their addresses and telephone numbers.

The content of such notification should state the facts as briefly and concisely as possible. If possible, mention of the names of individuals involved in the incident should be avoided. Since such notification can become a public record, open to use by the news media, care should be taken in its preparation in order to comply with existing regulations, but not to produce a severe public relations problem. Naturally, copies of any notification are a vital form of documentation and should be carefully kept as a permanent record.

H. Summary

A radiation emergency can occur wherever radioactive materials or radiation equipment are used, stored, or transported. Plans for the prompt notification and documentation of essential facts should be established as part of the radiation emergency procedure. The value of such preparedness for the possibility of a radiation accident, however remote it may seem, will provide the radiation user with protection against unnecessary risks to personnel and reputations. The value of proper documentation of a radiation accident should not be underestimated, and the legal requirements of reporting such accidents, within the prescribed reporting period, must not be overlooked. In the case of individuals potentially exposed as a result of an accident, it is just as important to document the absence of such exposure as it is to measure it accurately. The methods of obtaining documentation and preparation of the necessary reports are described. Certain recommendations are given for reducing the possible risks resulting from radiation accidents.

Appendix VI-1

EMERGENCY NOTIFICATION INSTRUCTIONS

These instructions are to be read and followed by all employees in the event of an emergency.

IMMEDIATE notification of an emergency is to be given by telephoning the following in numerical order:

FIRE

Organization or Individual		Telephone No.
1. ______ (location)	Fire Dept.	______
2. ______ (name)	RSO	______ (home)
3. ______		______

Information given by caller

1. Give your name.
2. Your company name.
3. Company address.
4. Location of fire.
5. Entrance firemen should use.
6. Caution if radioisotopes are involved.
7. Warn if airborne contamination "use masks".

1, 4, 5, 6, 7 - plus

(a) What has been done to control loss.

(b) When Fire Dept. was called.

(c) Current situation.

INJURY

1. Dr.______ ______ (office) ______ (office) ______ (home)

2. Dr.______ (alternate) ______ (office) ______ (office) ______ (home)

OR: Emergency Room______ (hospital)

3. ______ (company official) ______

Information given by caller

1. Extent of injury.
2. Present condition.
3. First aid measures taken.

ACCIDENTS

Organization or Individual	Telephone No.

1. If no injuries - no radiation,
   call: ______ (company official and title) ______

2. If radiation is involved,
   call: ______ (Radiation Safety Officer) ______ (home)

3. If accident occurred off-site, (e.g. on highway, etc.) have someone maintain security over radiation source and keep personnel away, while you call 'collect' the individuals named above - PLUS - highway patrol and/or police.

Information given by caller

1. What happened.
2. When.
3. Where.
4. Who was involved.
5. What has been done to control loss.
6. Current status.

Appendix VI-2

Radiation Incident Evaluation Record

In the event of a radiation accident, certain essential facts must be obtained as *promptly* and *accurately* as possible. These facts are needed to estimate the magnitude of the incident, limit the extent of damage, and institute remedial measures. *Remember,* try to obtain these facts calmly—use a recorder if possible. Be sure to note specific details on this sheet, including the *time* the information was received and the name of the person who furnished it.

Initial Incident Report	Response by	Time
1. What happened?		
2. When did it occur? (give time & date)		
3. Where did it happen? (building, floor, area)		
4. Who was involved? (names, employer)		
5. Who was exposed or injured? (name & the extent of injury or exposure)		
6. Where are the injured or exposed now?		
7. How much damage to facilities?		
(a). Was damage confined to company property?		
(b). What damage was done to property of others?		
8. Is radioactive contamination a problem?		
(a). If so, how extensive is contamination? (on-site, off-site?)		
(b). What is being done to control the contamination?		
9. Who, other than me, has been notified?		
10. Where can you be reached if we need you?		

Appendix VI-3

Preliminary Hazard Evaluation

1. Is outside help (fire, police, Atomic Energy Commission) required? If so, follow *Emergency Notification Instructions* (see Appendix VI-1).
2. Is medical assistance required?

3. Should personnel be evacuated:
   (a) From the incident area or building?
   (b) From the site?
   (c) From the locations off-site?
4. Has the *Radiation Emergency Plan* been activated?
   (a) Health Physics consultant notified?
   (b) If so, is additional help required?
   (c) Decontamination operations mobilized?
5. What is the accident classification?
6. Have official agencies been notified as required? (Atomic Energy Commission, state)
7. What are the immediate problems (off-site; on-site)?
8. What are the long-range problems (off-site; on-site)?
9. Estimate the duration of these problems (7 and 8).
10. Have the families of the injured been contacted?
11. What information should be given to the employees? By whom?
12. Has a newspaper release been prepared by company officials authorized to disseminate information to news media?

Appendix VI-4

FROM:__________________________
DATE: __________________________

MEMO TO:____________________________________
SUBJECT: INVESTIGATION OF RADIATION EXPOSURE

The objective of personnel radiation monitoring is to measure occupational radiation exposures and to aid in the detection of unnecessary radiation dosages. The prompt investigation of any above-average exposure will be useful in determining methods of preventing unnecessary radiation exposures from recurring.

During the period ____________________, your personnel radiation monitoring devices indicated an exposure of ____________________mR. The current permissible exposure level for x and gamma radiation is __________ __________mR/week.

Please answer the following questions and return this statement as quickly as possible so that our records may be properly evaluated.

1. How did the exposure occur?
2. Why did the exposure occur?
3. What has been done to prevent a recurrence of such an exposure?
4. Remarks

Signed____________________________________ Date____________
Employee

Forwarded____________________________________ Date____________
Supervisor

Appendix VI-5

A Suggested Checklist on

Radiation Accident Preparedness

The following items are some, but not necessarily all, of the essential points that should be considered when formulating an Emergency Plan. These items should be included in periodic evaluations of radiation users and their readiness for an emergency which, either directly or indirectly, may involve radiation. The current status of each item should be designated as satisfactory, marginal or unsatisfactory, and appropriate action should be taken to achieve the desired degree of protection.

Management — *Status (S, M, U*)*

1. Channel of command clearly established:
2. Emergency Procedures well defined and accepted:
3. Copy of Emergency Procedures on hand for key management personnel to use: (a) at office:
   (b) at home:
4. Communication channel established and posted:
   (a) Plan designates *who* to call *and* gives office and home telephone numbers.
   (b) Tells *what* information must be given.
   (c) Specifies a key employee as "information officer" authorized to cope with all official communications (e.g., news media) other than emergency calls.
5. Incident Evaluation Plan formulated and ready:
6. Damage Control Plan formulated and ready:
7. Medical Assistance Plan formulated and ready:
8. Incident Notification Plan formulated and ready:
9. Recovery Plan formulated and ready:

Health Physics; safety and security

1. Supervisors and radiation workers familiar with emergency procedures.
2. Copies of Emergency Procedures on hand at office and home.
3. Emergency Equipment and Instrumentation on "stand-by."
   a. Rescue equipment available and accessible.

Appendix VI-5 (Cont'd)

b. Portable instruments strategically stored.
c. Extra personnel monitoring equipment and protective clothing on "stand-by."

4. Channel of command clearly understood.
5. Emergency communications network planned and in readiness.
6. Radiation inventory current and radiation locations well defined.
7. Radiation Risk Evaluation Plans and data sheets formulated and ready.
8. Orientation on possible radiation emergencies given to:
   a. Supervisors and all radiation workers.
   b. Medical personnel to be called upon in an emergency.
   c. Local fire officials.
   d. Local police officials.
   e. Local public health officials.
9. In the event of an emergency (e.g., after hours) the above (8a to e) know *what* to do, *whom* to contact and *how* to cope with the incident as it pertains to their responsibilities.
10. Auxiliary personnel available to assist:
    a. Health physics.
    b. Medical.
    c. Security.
    d. Services (temporary power; procurement; communications).

Radiation Workers

1. Simplified Radiation Emergency Plan understood:
   a. Radiation warnings and alarms known.
   b. Evacuation signal and route known.
   c. Reassembly points (in safe area) specified.
2. Channels of Command clearly understood.
3. Damage Control Measures clearly stated.
4. Emergency Plan practiced at least once a year.
5. Each worker has received safety training relative to his radiological safety responsibilities and is familiar with the written operating procedures and regulations governing the routine and emergency conditions affecting his work.

Appendix VI-5 (Cont'd)

Medical Services

1. Availability of medical assistance for the types of potential injuries from this installation:
   (a) Specific physicians have reviewed potential injuries, including those which may involve radiation.
   (b) Plans are formulated and in readiness for:
      (1) Removal of injured to specific hospitals.
      (2) Notification of physician, emergency medical facilities.
2. Specific measures are to be taken to:
   (a) Provide prompt and effective medical aid for injured.
   (b) Control radiation risks to medical team.
   (c) Furnish radiation exposure evaluation data to physicians.
3. Key management and health physicists have established communication network (e.g., unlisted telephone numbers for emergency calls to hospital officials, physicians, etc.).
4. Adequate health physics assistance (certified health physicist or radiation physicist) is available should the physician require a consultation.

* S-Satisfactory; M-Marginal; U-Unsatisfactory

Appendix VI-6

Evaluation of Incidents or Occurrences Involving Radiation

	Accident Classification					
	For AEC Licensees (Per 10-CFR 20)			For AEC Operations (Per AEC Manual)		
	a	*b*	*c*	*A*	*B*	*C*
A. *Serious incident* involving radioactive materials or radiation producing equipment. *(Immediate notification required.)*						
1. For AEC Licensees and/or AEC Contractors:						
(a) Loss or theft of licensed radioactive material.	X			X		
(b) Exposure of individual's whole body to 25 rems or more.	X			X		
(c) Exposure of individual's skin of whole body to 150 rems or more.	X			X		
(d) Exposure of individual's hands/forearms, or feet/ankles to 375 rems or more.	X			X		
(e) Release of radioactive materials in concentrations which, if averaged over twenty-four hours, would exceed 5000 times the limits specified in Appendix B, Table II of Title 10-CFR-20.	X			X		
(f) Incident may result in loss of one or more work weeks of the operation of any facility.	X			X		
(g) Damage to property may exceed $100,000.	X			X		
2. In addition to the above, the following applies *only to* AEC installations and prime contractors:						
(a) Any incident involving an atomic weapon resulting in injury or damage to private property.				X		
(b) Any notice that an individual may have received 25 rems or more in a calendar year.				X		
(c) Any injury or illness diagnosed by a M.D. competent in nuclear medicine as having conceivably resulted from cumulative or massive radiation exposure.				X		
(d) Allegations that ex-employees of AEC or its contractors are disabled as a result of exposure to toxic materials or radiation related to atomic energy operations.				X		
(e) Any injury or industrial illness of five or more persons in AEC operation.				X		
(f) Any accident or radiation exposure which creates a significant public relations problem.				X		
(g) Any off-site accident involving vehicles carrying AEC shipments of radioactive materials.				X		

Appendix VI-6 (Cont'd)

	Accident Classification: For AEC Licensees (Per 10-CFR-20) *a*	*b*	*c*	For AEC Operations (Per AEC Manual) *A*	*B*	*C*
B. *Reportable accident (24 hour notification required)*						
(a) Exposure of individual's whole body to 5 rems or more.		X				
(b) Exposure of individual's skin of whole body to 30 rems or more.		X				
(c) Exposure of individual's hand/forearms or feet/ankles to 75 rems or more.		X				
(d) Release of radioactive materials in concentrations which, if averaged over twenty-four hours, would exceed 500 times the limits specified in the Appendix B, Table II, Title 10-CFR-20.		X				
(e) Incident may result in loss of one or more workdays of operation of any facility.		X				
(f) Property damage may exceed $1,000.		X				
(g) Incident may not result in any of the above, but may create serious public relations problems.		*				
(*NOTE—AEC does not *require* notification, but we suggest they be informed.)						
C. *Minor reportable occurrences (notification required within 30 days)*						
(a) Radiation exposure of any individual in excess of limits specified in 10-CFR-20 or AEC license conditions.			X			
(b) Radiation levels or radioisotope released in unrestricted areas which *have not* resulted in excessive exposures, but have been in excess of ten times any applicable limit set forth in 10-CFR-20 or the conditions specified in an AEC license.			X			
(c) Bodily injury, property damage or claim connected with the possession or use of radioactive material at a facility or in the course of transportation which would pertain to an indemnity agreement between the licensee and the AEC.			X			

Appendix VI-7

Radiation Incident Reporting Procedures

A. ***Reporting Type "A" Incidents:*** Require *IMMEDIATE* reports to U.S. Atomic Energy Commission, U.S. Department of Labor, and in certain states—to appropriate officials in the Health Department.

TYPE A-1

a) Immediately telephone the Director of the appropriate Atomic Energy Commission Regional Compliance Office listed in Appendix D of 10 CFR 20.

b) Confirm the telephone report with a telegram.

c) Within thirty days, the licensee must make a formal written report of the incident to the Director, Division of Licensing and Regulation, U.S. Atomic Energy Commission, Washington 25, D.C., with a copy to the Atomic Energy Commission Regional Compliance Office listed in Appendix D of 10 CFR 20.

d) We also recommend that the licensee maintain close liaison with the nearest Atomic Energy Commission Compliance Office by telephone during the first few days following discovery of the incident.

TYPE A-2

Refer to those requiring Atomic Energy Commission Contractors and Atomic Energy Commission installations to report *immediately* to the Atomic Energy Commission Headquarters responsible for these operations. Specific instructions are contained in Atomic Energy Commission Appendix 0502 of the Atomic Energy Commission's Operational Safety Handbook. These procedures do not apply to the average radioisotope licensee.

B. ***Reporting of Incidents Requiring Reports within 24 Hours:***

1) The licensee must notify the Director of the appropriate Atomic Energy Commission Division of Regional Compliance Office (see 10 CFR 20, Appendix D).

a) Within twenty-four hours after learning of an incident which may have caused, or threatens to cause, those effects listed in Part B, shall report as follows:

(1) Telephone the Atomic Energy Commission Director within twenty-four hours and report the incident.

(2) Confirm the telephone call by telegram within twenty-four hours.

(3) Provide a written report of the incident within thirty days to the Director of the Atomic Energy Commission Regional Compliance, Washington 25, D.C., with a copy to the appropriate Atomic Energy Commission Compliance Office. This written report must describe the extent of exposure, levels of concentrations, cause of exposure and corrective steps taken to avoid a recurrence.

C. ***Minor Incidents*** (Part C of Classification Outline) requires reports within thirty days. Report should be sent to the Director, Division of Licensing and Regulations, U.S. Atomic Energy Commission, Washington 25, D.C., with a copy to the appropriate Atomic Energy Commission Regional Compliance Office. This report must describe the extent of the exposures, levels of concentrations, cause of exposure and corrective measures taken to avoid recurrence.

D. ***Reporting "Type B" and "Type C" Incidents*** by Atomic Energy Commission Contractors and Atomic Energy Commission operations is specifically covered in the Atomic Energy Commission Manual, Appendix 0502, Parts II and III, and should be followed as necessary.

E. ***Other Accidents or Occurrences,*** which Atomic Energy Commission contractors must include in routine reports (also known as Type "C").

1) All accidents normally reported quarterly and annually.

2) Disabling occupational injuries.

3) Property damage or loss resulting from fires or other accidental causes.

4) All motor vehicle accidents (government vehicles only).

REFERENCES

1. Code of Federal Regulations. Title 10, Atomic Energy; Part 20, Standards for Protection Against Radiation. *Federal Register,* U.S. Government Printing Office, Washington, D.C., November 17, 1960.
2. Code of Federal Regulations. The Walsh-Healy Act. *Federal Register,* U.S. Government Printing Office, Washington, D.C., (in press).
3. *Reporting and Investigating Accidents and Radiation Exposures.* Division of Operational Safety, U.S. Atomic Energy Commission Manual, Appendix 0502, U.S. Government Printing Office, Washington, D.C., April 4, 1962.
4. Saenger, E. L., ed.: *Medical Aspects of Radiation Accidents.* U.S. Government Printing Office, Washington, D.C., 1963.
5. Brodsky, A., and Beard, G. V.: *A Compendium of Information for Use in Controlling Radiation Emergencies.* U.S. Atomic Energy Commission, U.S. Government Printing Office, Washington, D.C., February 1960.
6. *Exposure to Radiation in an Emergency.* National Committee on Radiation Protection and Measurements, Report No. 29, Section of Nuclear Medicine, The University of Chicago, Chicago, Illinois, January 1962.

EMERGENCY PLANS AT UNIVERSITIES

PAUL L. ZIEMER
Bionucleonics Department
Purdue University
Lafayette, Indiana

THE GROWING CONCERN for radiation emergency planning is particularly pertinent in view of the rapid growth of the nuclear industry and the increased utilization of radiation and radioactivity. This increased utilization is reflected in our university programs just as it is in industry and in medicine. Of the eighty-six licenses first issued by the U.S. Atomic Energy Commission in 1946, twenty-two went to universities and colleges (1). This number has grown until, today, there are over 400 universities and colleges listed by the Atomic Energy Commission as possessing byproduct material licenses (2). This does not include other types of university facilities such as reactors and x-ray devices.

Diversity of Radiation Utilization in the University

Before discussing particular aspects of university emergency plans, let us consider the structure of radiation programs in universities. Wide variations may exist in universities and colleges with respect to types and levels of radiation in use, applications of the radiation, and details of protection programs. For example, a university may have a very limited isotope or radiation program, perhaps under an individual specific license; or it may have a large-scale program under a broad license, or even elaborate reactor and irradiation facilities. The health physics programs in universities may be handled variously by student health services, offices of environmental health and safety, or simply by a radiation safety committee (3). Thus, it is not possible to make statements which will apply equally to all universities; but some general statements can be made which will be applicable in most cases.

In the university situation, normal diversity of interest in the various departments usually leads to a radiation and radioisotope program which is very broad and varied, involving multiple uses and applications of radiation. The program is actually a composite of those found in industry, research, medicine, agriculture, and government agencies. For example, at Purdue University there are low-level tracer laboratories, high-level irradiation facilities, low-level teaching laboratories, accelerators of all types, sealed sources, a reactor, an exponential pile, x-ray facilities, thickness and density gauges, and medical diagnostic facilities (medical applications at Purdue include treatment of animals in the school of veterinary medicine).

The wide variety of radiation sources found in universities is a natural consequence of the university fulfilling its functions of teaching and research in many fields of interest. As a result, the potential exists for a great variety of radiation emergencies, with respect to types of radiation as well as levels. The university health physicist must be prepared to cope with problems and emergencies involving essentially all aspects of radiation research, instruction, and utilization.

It is also likely that the university will find itself in a position of having sources of radiation distributed over a rather large number of buildings throughout the campus and not conveniently located in a single building. This becomes an important factor in emergency planning, with respect to communications as well as to location of emergency equipment.

The University Health Physics Program

University radioisotope programs are usually carried out under "broad" U.S. Atomic Energy Commission byproduct material licenses (or the equivalent in those states in which an agreement between the federal government and the state is in effect). Under the terms of such licenses, it is necessary to have a functioning radioisotope committee. Committee members should be of a high staff level, preferably of professorial rank; they should be competent in training and experience and able to evaluate all aspects of radiation safety problems.

It would seem prudent for the university to establish a single committee to handle the over-all radiation safety program under powers more inclusive than required for U.S. Atomic Energy Commission licensing—that is, the committee's responsibility should extend to all radiation hazards including x-rays and radium. If other committees, such as a reactor safeguards committee or a human use committee, are needed, they could function as subcommittees of the main radiation safety committee. This would provide a means of co-ordinating all the radiation safety programs on the campus. The radioisotope or radiation safety committee should be free or independent of any particular school or department in the university, being perhaps a committee of the president or the vice-president.

The university health physics group operates under the policies established by the radiation safety committee, but may itself be a part of some particular department such as student health, radiology, environmental sanitation, or campus safety. Health physics constitutes a separate team in the university from medical or security groups, even though it may functionally be in the same department as one of these. This fact, however, does not preclude the close liaison of health physics with these other groups.

Team Planning in University Emergencies

Most universities have their own safety and security forces or campus police. Many have their own fire departments. All have a medical staff of some sort, either in a student hospital, health center, or the medical school. In emergency planning, the health physics team must work closely with safety, fire, and medical personnel in order to co-ordinate the activities of these groups and to acquaint them with particular hazards in the various areas of the campus. For example, safety and security personnel, including the fire department, should be provided with basic information as to the location (building and room) of radiation and radioisotope areas, as well as information on special precautions wherever indicated. Short courses to acquaint staff police and firemen with radiation and health physics fundamentals are in order as well.

Major campus buildings often have their own safety subcommittees which help to carry out normal departmental safety programs under the over-all campus safety program. Health physics activities and emergency plans should be co-ordinated with these safety subcommittees whenever possible.

Most universities have a news bureau or information bureau which handles news releases for the institution. This is the logical place through which to channel information in an emergency. At Purdue University, for example, the Bureau of Information is part of the present emergency organization. Any inquiries made to emergency personnel, such as police, fire, medical, or health physics teams, are referred directly to the Bureau which, in turn, clears its releases through the university administration.

Universities are very much conscious of money and economics, and the remarks by Dr. Whipple (see page 225) with respect to developing a program which is economically feasible are quite applicable to the university situation. Thus, realistic emergency planning indicates that there are certainly some areas in the university which require only a minimum of basic general instructions for emergencies, whereas the higher-level facilities may require detailed written plans of action and appropriate emergency equipment. An initial analysis of each area prior to the initiation of radioisotope or radiation work enables the health physics group to place emergency procedure emphasis in the most important areas.

Emergency Planning and the University Population

Emergency planning must take into account the types of individuals involved, particularly with respect to their knowledge of radiation hazards, as well as the physical factors of the facility. A large proportion of the radiation work in a university, both in teaching and in research, is carried out directly by professorial staff at the doctorate level. The rest of the workers are students, primarily graduate students, and technicians. Almost without exception, these individuals are quite well trained in using radiation and radioisotopes. This fact can be very helpful in minimizing hazards. When emergencies do arise, these individuals can be of assistance to the health physicist and may actually make up part of an emergency team in a given area.

There may, however, also be some disadvantages involved in relying on these individuals. I have seen cases where doctorate-level personnel were not willing to admit inability to cope with certain situations, and delays in notifying the health physics staff of the emergency resulted. Thus, it is important that emergency plans stress promptness in reporting anything suspicious, even though false alarms may occasionally result.

If an emergency does arise on campus, the university may find itself in a rather delicate position due to the presence of students on the campus. Emergency plans must take into consideration the fact that large groups of students may be in the vicinity at the time an emergency arises. Proper handling of publicity is very important at this point, since parents of students will be greatly concerned about the safety of their sons and daughters and may have to rely on the various news media for information.

The University's Role in Emergency Training

Since the university's main job is to train, instruct, and teach people, it seems reasonable that students learning to work with radiation should also learn how to formulate emergency plans as part of their training. In fact, the university may not be fulfilling its function if it simply hands a student a set of emergency plans and says, "Here is what to do in case of an emergency." Rather, it is worthwhile whenever possible to have students and staff who work in a given radioisotope or radiation area work up emergency plans for their area. These plans should then be submitted to the health physicist and the radiation safety committee for review. Suggestions and modifications will often be necessary, but the end result is not only a plan that is well thought out, but one with which the workers themselves are intimately familiar. Their own responsibilities as well as those of the emergency team will be clearly defined in their minds. As a byproduct of this process, the student will be better prepared to go out into industry, government, or education and to utilize such training.

Reporting of Incidents

The university, like any other institution, is responsible for reporting accidents or incidents involving radiation to an appropriate government agency. In the case of U.S. Atomic Energy Commission licensees, the Atomic Energy Commission's regional office is the appropriate agency to which the report must be submitted. In some cases, reporting to a state agency is required, particularly in the states which have assumed the Atomic Energy Commission licensing function. Such reporting should be the designated responsibility of the radiation safety committee or of the health physics staff.

Within the institution itself, reports of incidents must be made directly to the health physics emergency staff. Thus, in each laboratory or radiation facility there must be posted in a prominent place, preferably near the phone, the office and home phone numbers of the health physics team, police and fire departments, and physicians. Since graduate students and even staff members in the university often find it necessary to carry out research at all hours of the day and night, the health physics team must be on twenty-four hour call.

Experience at Purdue indicates that most emergencies in the university tend to be rather minor. This, of course, does not preclude the possibility of major emergencies. In the last fifteen years, only two incidents have occurred at Purdue for which reporting to the Atomic Energy Commission was required. One case involved a fire which broke out near, but not in an isotope laboratory. The emergency personnel and firemen who were called to the scene became concerned about possible radiation hazards and called on the health physics group for assistance. Although no radiation or contamination problems were involved, it turned out that there was a monetary loss in the radioisotope laboratory as a result of smoke damage. This laboratory, being under a slight negative pressure, drew in the smoke from the nearby fire through the louvers in the door, which led to smoke and soot damage of all of the equipment in the room. Because of the monetary loss, the incident was reported to the Atomic Energy Commission.

The second case involved a cobalt-60 irradiator whose 800-curie source was found to be leaking. Although no contamination of personnel and equipment resulted, reporting of the incident was required under the conditions of the sealed-source license.

Other emergencies have been minor, due primarily to the low level of activity in use. Nevertheless, even minor emergencies should be treated with concern in the university, inasmuch as a conservative approach is appropriate for training staff and students in emergency procedures. Thus, at Purdue, even a minor emergency involves reporting of the incident in full to the university radioisotope committee and to departmental administrators. Reports are also required from the individuals involved as to corrective measures which will be taken in the future to prevent reoccurrence of the incident.

Summary

Work with radiation and radioisotopes in the university covers a broad spectrum of kinds, levels, and applications. Thus, emergencies of every conceivable type must be anticipated. Use of the team approach involving the coordinated efforts of health physics, security, fire, medical, and publicity personnel is suggested. Professorial staff and graduate students with training in radioisotope handling techniques should be considered for providing assistance whenever possible. Furthermore, the health physics staff should make every effort to involve the research personnel directly in the formulation of emergency plans for their respective areas.

REFERENCES

1. *Radioisotopes in Science and Industry.* A Special Report of the U.S. Atomic Energy Commission, U.S. Government Printing Office, Washington, D.C., p. 100, January 1960.
2. *Major Activities in the Atomic Energy Programs, January-December, 1962.* U.S. Atomic Energy Commission, U.S. Government Printing Office, Washington, D.C., p. 578, January 1963.
3. Prince, John R.: Radiation Safety in a University. *Health Physics, 9*:347-349, 1963.

DISCUSSION

Mr. A. Weintraub (U.S. Atomic Energy Commission, Health and Safety Laboratory) : I have two comments. In relation to the possibility of spread of contamination by firefighters, I think there is a great oversight here. The fire department should be brought in long before the emergency exists. There should be a pre-fire planning association with the fire department so that they know exactly what is on the scene and so that they will be prepared before the incident occurs.

Dr. Whipple referred to a manual that might be too binding. This is a very real problem, and we solved this in New York, I believe, by giving the field commander the greatest latitude. We give him guidelines. We don't tell him exactly what he can do. We have enough faith in our team captains so that we know they will probably do the right thing if we don't bind them in the manual.

In relation to the number of team members that were noted by Dr. Whipple, there is one who, I think, ranks with the top, who was left out, and that is the public information officer. Most of the incidents that have occurred have led to the greatest damage in the fact that the public communications media do not get the correct information, that they overemphasize or give the wrong information. I think that, if we had a public information officer, or perhaps one of the other team members you enumerated, trained to give information properly, this would contribute greatly toward keeping these emergencies in their proper perspective.

Mr. R. G. Gallaghar: I think your remarks and comments are quite well taken. We can't urge too strongly that any installation that has radioisotopes or even radiation-producing equipment have a session with the fire marshal. They are intelligent men who generally handle a situation expertly. They deplore being left out of your planning.

Dr. G. H. Whipple: In reply to the statement attributed to me, I express my gratification. With regard to the public relations man, I wonder if the gentleman was thinking perhaps of a larger installation than I was trying to include in my remarks. There are many fairly good-sized radioactive facilities that would find it very awkward indeed to keep a public relations man on tap twenty-four hours a day. I would presume that the management position, the first one I mentioned in my key spots in the emergency organization, perhaps would cover this. Where you have a large enough installation, you always count on getting the public relations man out of bed sober and alert.

Mr. R. G. Gallaghar: In several instances, the lack of a specified management individual who is a spokesman for the company has created headlines, embarrassing ones, because they didn't relate in a factual way to the incident. Thus, in planning, it is essential that, immediately following an incident, employees again be reminded that the company or organization will have any statement to the public press made through one individual. He will make it factual and informative; any other statements are not only out of line and should be avoided, but also could be a detriment to the reputation of the firm and actually risk the employees' jobs in the radiation installation.

Chairman C. M. Patterson: I am told that one organization has a set of ready-made comments for the press before management or a public relations officer may get to the scene, and he just has to pull the right envelope from among twenty or so and there is your press release.

Mr. T. N. Hubbard (University of Alabama): Since we are getting down to specifics today, I think we ought to talk about incidents, particularly with regard to firemen, and I throw this out only as a suggestion. We have some forty firemen in the city of Tuskaloosa, Alabama, and I have given at least three hours of indoctrination and training to all these firemen. I don't think we can overemphasize this.

Also, in case of a fire, I don't think you should bind the firemen in any respect. I have given our fire department a listing of all the locations of the radioactive sources within the University of Alabama by building and room number, and I have also categorized them—the lower-energy radioisotopes, in microcurie amounts generally. I have told them in each instance of fire to contact me, but in dealing with lower levels of radioisotopes, I have told them to go ahead and deal with the fire and contact me as soon as they can.

Also, I think it is very important that we deal with the police as well as the firemen.

I just want to point these areas out in that I want them to notify me, but I want them to deal with the situation as well, and I don't want to give them too much instruction.

Dr. A. A. Spritzer (University of Pittsburgh): I'd like to make a suggestion to those people responsible for setting up your training manuals and procedures not to forget the hospital aspects in your procedures. In our experience, at least, even those installations that have very thorough emergency plans tend to forget that one aspect of the planned emergency procedures involves what I refer to as disposition of patients. Now, this can take many forms, either in secondary control areas, at home, or what not, or holding patients for medical surveillance, but one specific form is disposition to a hospital, and I would therefore suggest that you consider having the hospital emergency plan incorporated as an appendix into your own plant emergency procedures, to make sure that there is a fair degree of integration between the two facilities.

Chairman C. M. Patterson: I have been quite interested in hearing about public relations and training and all the comments that have been made, and I'd like to relate one instance in north Georgia where a nuclear facility was installed. The company which was operating this facility went to considerable effort in educating the public. They hired people who went around to the PTA, the Kiwanis Club, Lions, etc., trying to educate the natives of north Georgia about the problems of radiation and what kind of neighbor they were going to be, and that they were really a good neighbor. The most interesting thing that developed was that these hill people thought this was going to lead to certain mutations and genetic occurrences, and that there was a 2,000-pound rat devastating the countryside. This story got started. All of us see the humor in a story like this; but in certain quarters of north Georgia they actually believed it.

Mr. F. R. Jordan (Rock Island Arsenal, Rock Island, Illinois): I am one of the fire chiefs here in the room. I would just like to comment that it really is very important to the firefighters that information be given to us. Now, a lot of fire departments carry a 5 x 7 card in their car or in their emergency equipment, which not only would give information on handling a nuclear incident, but which are indexed with the pre-fire plan for each individual building we might have in the locality.

Mr. R. G. Gallaghar: Naturally, any emergency situation can help you gain some form of experience to help you face another emergency, and in connection with notifying the proper superior, I'd like to relate one story that occurred in the South Pacific.

There was a very notorious Navy pilot who really hadn't done a thing in combat, and the rest of his buddies were upset about him. One day he decided to make amends, so he took off from a Navy carrier, flew high over the Pacific, looked down, saw a Japanese submarine, zoomed down, dropped a depth charge and blew up the submarine. He roared up again, looked around, and there was a tender that had been servicing the sub. He zoomed down, dropped a charge and blew up the tender. Then he saw a Jap shore installation, and blew up an ammunition dump. He came out of his run in time to see a Zero, but he was out of ammunition. Looking down, he saw the flight deck, and made a beautiful landing on the carrier. He said, "Well, Skipper, I had a beautiful day. I sank a sub, a tender, and blew up an ammunition dump. What do you think of that for a day?" A voice came, "Oh, so, velly good day. You make only one mistake—wrong carrier!" So, notification must be to the proper official.

Mr. F. L. Bordell (Westinghouse Atomic Power): Dr. Forgotson, you mentioned that juries are involved. Do all radiation cases, that is, lawsuits, have to go before a jury?

Dr. E. H. Forgotson: Well, the answer to that is "no." If they are common law cases, they would go to a jury. If it is workmen's compensation, they may or may not go to a jury, depending on the jurisdiction involved, and if the case comes under the Federal Tort Claims Act against the U.S. Government, it would be ruled on by a judge. In any case, there would be a fact-finding by a person or persons who might not necessarily have expert medical or health physics knowledge.

Mr. T. Fields: Akin to the remarks by Dr. Whipple and Dr. Ziemer about selection of personnel, I might make a remark about an incident that actually did happen in our hospital within the last few months.

We have a limited number of health physics personnel there, and of course, when anything does happen, such as a spill, we impress the person responsible for it into the labor pool for cleaning it up. This happened to a girl chemist, and of course she was obliged to help us scrub up the floors and everything else. When I got home that night, I got a rather excited call from the director of the hospital. It turned out that the girl was his daughter, and I had to give him a rather thorough lecture on the hazards of cleaning up a radioactive spill.

Dr. P. L. Ziemer: Let me make a comment on that. We do not use any janitorial service at all for cleaning up spills. With a spill, usually the person responsible cleans it up, or if not, it is cheaper to use graduate students than janitors.

Mr. J. Novak (Argonne National Laboratory): Have you ever run across a problem of exposure of individuals under eighteen years of age at the university, and how do you handle that?

Dr. P. L. Ziemer: Well, of course, there are exposure limits for individuals under eighteen years of age, namely, 10 per cent of the stated limits. Most of our work with radioisotopes involves graduate students. They are generally over eighteen. We have had cases where undergraduates may have been involved at very low levels of radioactivity. These were perhaps senior students, and they could be individuals of seventeen, or conceivably younger. However, it is really only an academic question, at least in our situation, since we never have had any regular personnel who have approached normal exposure limits.

Mr. R. L. Clark (Nuclear—Chicago): Dr. Ziemer, in the accident which you had, you cleaned up the smoke damage which I assume was not due to contamination. Suppose you had decided not to clean this up; therefore you wouldn't have spent the money. Obviously, then, you wouldn't have had to report it. Is that correct?

Dr. P. L. Ziemer: When the fire occurred, we didn't have any idea whether we would be in a situation in which we would have to make a report; therefore, to be on the safe side, we reported. Whenever there is a question as to whether or not to report, it would seem to me that it is the prudent thing to do.

Mr. R. L. Clark: Did you do this on your own, or did someone say you had to report?

Dr. P. L. Ziemer: No, we had to make a decision as to whether we believed this was a point where we came under 10 CFR 20* regulation on reporting. We were not certain at that point what the dollar value of the damage done in the room would be, so we reported, to be on the safe side.

*Code of Federal Regulations, Title 10, Atomic Energy, Part 20. Copies are available from the nearest U.S. Atomic Energy Commission licensing authority.

Chapter VII

GOVERNMENT SERVICES AND REGULATIONS

FEDERAL RADIATION COUNCIL PROTECTION GUIDES

CLAIRE C. PALMITER
Federal Radiation Council
Washington, D.C.

I WANT TO present to you some history of the formation of the Federal Radiation Council, note its reports, discuss some of the applications of its radiation protection guidance recommendations, and finally tell you of some of its proposed activities for the immediate future.

The Federal Radiation Council was established by Executive Order 10831 on August 14, 1959, and was made statutory by Public Law 86-373 on September 23, 1959, as an amendment to the Atomic Energy Act of 1954. The Executive Order was the culmination of a special study on the problem of radiation protection, particularly as related to fallout resulting from the testing of nuclear weapons, conducted by the Director of the Bureau of the Budget; the Chairman of the U.S. Atomic Energy Commission; and the Secretary of Health, Education, and Welfare.

In the period immediately preceding the issuance of the Executive Order, the position of the Atomic Energy Commission was becoming increasingly difficult because of its dual responsibility, under the Atomic Energy Act, of promoting the uses of nuclear technology on the one hand, and of simultaneously protecting public health and safety on the other. The creation of the Federal Radiation Council was the Government's answer to this problem. Under the terms of PL 86-373, "The Council shall advise the President with respect to radiation matters, directly or indirectly affecting health, including guidance for all Federal agencies in the formulation of radiation standards and in the establishment and execution of programs of cooperation with States."

The rationale presented in the supporting documents recognized quite clearly that, when programs of nuclear technology are established in the national interest, and when these necessitate exposure of the general public, the whole problem of the balance between the need for the program on the one hand and the possible effects on the health of the public on the other involves fundamental decisions on public policy influencing national security, economics, industry, labor, and many equally important ramifications of our national existence.

Since such judgments are political decisions, in the highest sense of the word, it was determined that the President should be advised on such matters by the highest political appointees with responsibilities on the subject in the Executive Branch of the Government. The present composition of the Federal Radiation Council, accordingly, consists of the Secretary of Health, Education, and Welfare, who is its present Chairman; the Chairman of the Atomic Energy Commission; Secretary of Defense; Secretary of Commerce; Secretary of Labor; and the Secretary of Agriculture. The President's Science Adviser is authorized to attend the Council meetings and take part in its deliberations. It is appropriate, I believe, to note that Dr. Jerome Wiesner, acting in this capacity, was a very influential contributor to the activities of the Federal Radiation Council.

The first meeting of the Council was devoted to a consideration of its internal organization and a "White Paper" on radiation. The Executive Order provided for Council agencies to assign employees to the Council; Dr. Donald R. Chadwick, presently Chief of the Division of Radiological Health, U.S. Public Health Service, was detailed to the position of Council Secretary. In August, 1960, I was assigned from the Atomic Energy Commission to the Council staff. At the first meeting, the decision was made to vest the operating responsibility for the Council activities in a Working Group composed of senior technical representatives from each of the constituent agencies on the Council. This Working Group, with the assistance of the Staff and consultants, was responsible for the development of the Council program, technical review of documents, and the formulation of recommendations for Council consideration and approval.

Thus, the Federal Radiation Council, which is itself a Cabinet-level special committee, established an internal "government by committee" with both the strengths and frustrations that this statement implies. The strength lies in the view that, where matters of such fundamental policy are concerned, it is important that recommendations being made to the President represent a true consensus of the operating agencies which have responsibilities in the field. The weaknesses, such as they are, might be described by the usual facetious description that "a camel is a horse put together by a committee." The activities of the Federal Radiation Council during the past have reflected both attributes of its internal organization.

By the time the Federal Radiation Council began to function, the voluntary moratorium on weapons testing that occurred after the cessation of the testing programs in 1958 was in being, and the preoccupation with fallout tended to diminish. As an outgrowth of the "White Paper," mentioned previously, the first report of the Federal Radiation Council covering radiation protection guidance for Federal agencies was issued in May 1960. The related Memorandum which contained seven recommendations was approved by the President on May 13, 1960. Both the Memorandum and the Report pointed out that there can be no single permissible or acceptable level of exposure without regard to the reason for permitting the exposure, and that, as a general principle, *radiation protection guidance involves a continuous balance between benefits and risks.*

Report No. 1 defined and provided Radiation Protection Guides (RPG's) for workers in occupations which arise in normal peacetime operations. For an individual in the population, an annual whole-body RPG of 0.5 rem and a thirty-year average gonadal dose of 5 rem was established. The Memorandum also stated that "The Radiation Protection Guides provide a general framework for the radiation protection requirements. It is expected that each Federal agency, by virtue of its immediate knowledge of its operating problems, will use these Guides as a basis upon which to develop detailed standards to meet its particular requirements."

The issuance of this report was greeted with a barrage of questions on the Federal Radiation Council's definition of "normal peacetime operations" and the interpretation of the "escape clause" that some people saw in Recommendation 7 of the accompanying Memorandum for the President, which was:

> "The Federal agencies apply these Radiation Protection Guides with judgment and discretion, to assure that reasonable probability is achieved in the attainment of the desired goal of protecting man from the undesirable effects of radiation. The Guides may be exceeded only after the Federal agency having jurisdiction over the matter has carefully considered the reasons for doing so in light of the recommendations in this paper."

The second report of the Federal Radiation Council, also devoted to Radiation Protection Guides for normal peacetime operations, was issued in September, 1961. The related Memorandum was approved by the President on September 21, 1961. Report No. 2 provided additional Radiation Protection Guides for individuals in the population for the particular organs, thyroid, bone marrow, and bone. In addition, these basic Radiation Protection Guides were translated to an equivalent daily intake of the specific nuclides, iodine-131, strontium-90, strontium-89, and radium-226, which would be expected to lead to an annual dose that can be compared with the Radiation Protection Guide for the corresponding organ.

Recognizing the transient nature of the appearance of radionuclides in the environment and the uneven distribution between different components of the diet, three general ranges of intake were provided and related to three different scales of action. These were labeled Ranges I, II, and III. The action specified in Report No. 2 when annual concentrations for radionuclides in the environment corresponding to Range III were encountered for normal peacetime operations was: "evaluation and application of additional control measures as necessary."

The Union of Soviet Socialist Republics broke the testing moratorium in September, 1961, by conducting an intensive atmospheric testing program. The Federal Radiation Council immediately addressed its attention to a review of all the current information regarding the inventories of radionuclides in the environment, as well as population exposures resulting from the testing of nuclear devices, and evaluated the possible range of biological effects that might conceivably be associated with such exposures. The report covering these studies was issued in May, 1962, as Federal Radiation Council Report No. 3, "Health Implications of Fallout from Nuclear Weapons Testing Through 1961."

The testing programs of 1961 and 1962 were attended by the rapid appearance of iodine-131 in the food supplies of this country, and by early 1962, cumulative levels for the annual intake of radioactive iodine in some sections of the country were approaching the top of Range II as specified by Report No. 2.

It was becoming abundantly clear by the time of the Joint Committee on Atomic Energy hearings on *Radiation Standards, Including Fallout,* conducted in May 1962, that the Federal Radiation Council had, indeed, created a camel with at least two humps, and that both of them were legitimate parts of the horse. One hump said that the guides did apply to fallout and that health protection agencies were expected to take such action as was necessary to insure that the annual consumption of iodine-131 did not exceed the top of Range II. This interpretation of the intent of the report was widely adopted by many people and agencies whose primary responsibility is health protection.

The other hump said that the numerical values for iodine-131 set up in Report No. 2 were designed to control normal peacetime operations of a continuing nature and were, therefore, predicated on radiation exposure levels that could readily be tolerated for a lifetime without any substantive effect on the health of the people concerned. Therefore, it did not appear reasonable to interpret the numerical values given in Report No. 2 as stipulating the conditions under which environmental controls had to be instituted for health protection purposes from an intermittent transient source such as that represented by the testing of nuclear weapons.

In this interpretation, the instruction for "evaluation and application of additional control measures as necessary" meant that the source of the iodine, its probable frequency of appearance, and the top levels that it might reasonably be expected to reach should be considered, and a specific medical evaluation made as to the probable health consequences from such conditions.

However, the numerical values of Report No. 2 by this view simply could not be used to indicate either when or what kind of protective action might be needed in response to environmental contamination such as that associated with fallout from the testing of nuclear weapons.

It is important to realize that these two humps of the camel represent differences in the basic philosophy for coping with environmental hazards. Each has far-reaching implications regarding Presidential decisions concerned with national security, economics, food and agriculture, distribution and use of food, and many equally serious ramifications of our national life.

During the past 18 months the Council has, through press releases, letters to Congress, etc., taken the following steps:

1) It has specifically denied the applicability of existing Radiation Protection Guides as illustrated in Reports 1 and 2 as being entirely relevant to decisions concerned with fallout.

2) It has established a basis for defining "normal peacetime operations" as those activities of a routine, continuing scientific, and industrial nature which are, or may be, subject to regulation.

3) Both Reports 1 and 2 are guides for administrative control purposes and cannot be extended to any other activity, and

4) No definitive guide, or guidance, has been adopted for application to any activity not fitting this definition.

In short, the Council, through a process of evolution, has faced squarely up to the fact that concepts, techniques, and procedures which are perfectly appropriate for industrial health protection cannot be extrapolated verbatim to other kinds of activities such as those represented by the atmospheric testing of nuclear weapons, the testing of peaceful uses of nuclear explosives, space applications, nuclear-powered aircraft and rockets, and similar ongoing development programs which either are being or have been actively pursued by the Federal Government. Other gaps in the available armament include the old problem of appropriate criteria, techniques, and procedures for coping with possible radiation accidents in which public exposure is a consideration; I shall say more about this later.

Commencing in August, 1962, the Council reexamined its internal organization and decided that it would do its job better if it had a full-time permanent professional staff, albeit a small one, hired by the Council and responsible to the Council rather than to any single member agency. Thereupon, the Chairman appointed a subcommittee consisting of one representative each from the Department of Health, Education, and Welfare; from the Atomic Energy Commission; and from the staff of the President's Science Adviser, to make recommendations for a permanent staff, determine what budgetary adjustments would have to be made to accommodate this change, and report back to the Council. This study was conducted from September, 1962, to February, 1963.

At its meeting in February, 1963, the Council decided that it wanted a staff which would be administratively and technically accountable directly to the Council for the documents and papers to be considered by the Council. An Executive Director was to have full operating responsibility, from the viewpoint of seeking necessary consultation, to get the technical backing for any recommendations, to isolate and identify the underlying policy problems on which the Council members would have to act, and to insure that the Council had access to the necessary supporting staff work to make a reasonable evaluation of the implications of available alternatives.

Dr. Paul C. Tompkins was appointed in March of 1963 by the U.S. Atomic Energy Commission to serve in the capacity of Acting Executive Director while the administrative machinery was getting organized. During the latter part of September, both of us were transferred permanently to the Council. Such a small staff, of course, could not be expected to stand by itself on all matters of concern to the Council. As noted in the statute forming the Council, "it shall consult qualified scientists and experts in radiation matters, including the President of the National Academy of Sciences, the Chairman of the National Committee on Radiation Protection and Measurements, and qualified experts in the fields of biology and medicine and in the field of health physics." We have done this in the past on many occasions, and recently have taken steps to formalize our relationships with the National Academy of Sciences and the National Committee on Radiation Protection and Measurements.

Under this reorganization, the first project activated was the preparation of a report updating FRC Report No. 3, taking into account the nuclear testing programs which had been conducted by both the United States and the Union of Soviet Socialist Republics in 1962. It was also evident that the Federal Radiation Council, as the obvious government spokesman on this subject, should be prepared to present to the President a unified government evaluation of the health implications to be anticipated from these series.

All of the interested agencies immediately assigned technical experts to a Council *ad hoc* panel which was set up to prepare the report.

Thanks to the admirable cooperation of everyone concerned, and a "few hours of night oil," such an evaluation was pulled together and approved by the White House. It was issued as Federal Radiation Council Report No. 4, "Estimates and Evaluation of Fallout in the United States from Nuclear Weapons Testing Conducted Through 1962," in time for discussion at this year's hearings by the Joint Committee on Atomic Energy.

Chapter 6 of this report, the Evaluation Section, quite clearly reflects the view that, although decision making has not been relegated to compliance with numbers in this field, it is still possible to insure that the public health is adequately protected when the machinery exists for quantitatively evaluating the magnitude of the anticipated challenge (that is, prediction of fallout levels) and, on the basis of this information, rendering a specific judgment regarding the need for health protection actions by responsible health authorities.

All of the Government statements presented to the Joint Committee in Phase I of the hearings, *Fallout, Radiation Standards, and Countermeasures,* conducted early last June, were presented under the auspices of the Federal Radiation Council. This, to my mind, is the most significant activity in which the Council has been involved during the past year.

The whole subject of fallout from the 1962 test program, predictions of quantities to be expected in food supplies and the whole gamut of considerations which must go into any reasonable approach to the problem of instituting health protection or control actions on the basis of environmental radionuclide levels, was gone into at great length.

The period from March through July 1963 was devoted entirely to the technical problems inherent in the compilation of Report No. 4, the preparation of testimony to be given to the Joint Committee in June, and several activities which were associated with the wind-up, so to speak, of Government participation in these hearings. Much of what I have said about the Council's technical activities during the past year is either stated or strongly implied by the record of the hearings.

The result was that the Council: a) acknowledged the nonexistence of guides applicable to the initiation of public health control actions related to fallout and environmental radioactivity, and b) accepted a commitment to have definitive proposals relative to this subject available within a year. This means approximately May, 1964.

Now I should like to discuss some of the important aspects which will have to be considered in formulating any proposals on this subject. Many activities involving exposure to radiation can be conducted with acceptable risks to health and safety. The problem is, to determine what risks are to be considered acceptable under particular sets of circumstances. Contrary to an opinion which is frequently held, the answer cannot be given on the basis of health considerations alone. If there were no reasons for accepting some degree of risk, health considerations would suggest *no* exposure to radiation. Nor can one determine a level of exposure of which he can say that smaller exposures are of little concern, but above which exposure to radiation really becomes dangerous. As far as can be determined, when levels of exposure increase, there is no level at which a small increase in exposure involves a large or abrupt increase in risk.

However, for wise planning and for administrative use in case of a radiation emergency, both on an industrial basis and for effecting countermeasures in the event of radioactive fallout, *there is need, before the incident, of a series of dose-effect tables relating biological effects to different types and levels of exposure conditions.* As is noted in the paper by Keene *et al.* in the Health Physics Journal, Volume 9, (No. 8), August 1963:

> "Maximum personnel doses appropriate to various types of emergency action should be determined in advance, and working limits established with due recognition of the fact that the probability and the seriousness of measurement errors may be abnormally high under emergency conditions. Where possible, "go, no go" type criteria should be pre-established, with consideration given to the urgency of the work, the dose rates encountered, the time required to complete the mission, and the relative benefits and risks involved in the successful completion of the mission."

Quoting also from the paper by Dr. Pochin given at the Hanford Symposium on the Biology of Radioiodine, ". . . the doses that may be received under accidental conditions seem like an argument as to how soon after the horse has gone the stable door should be shut. An accidental dose limit, however, has meaning if, but only if it is related to some remedial measure to prevent the dose from going even higher. It is not, therefore, dependent upon any simple balance between the hazard involved from radiation and, for example, the probability of the accident, but upon whether the risks involved in a practicable remedial measure are greater or less than the risks of allowing the radiation exposure to continue or increase. As in all the other instances we have reviewed, one may here again be faced with the balancing of incommensurables. Would you rather have ten road accidents while distributing dried milk or one possibly treatable thyroid cancer twenty years later? Is it preferable to move the aged and infirm 100 miles by road or to subject them to 50 rad from a continuing environmental contamination? The level at which one applies the remedy may depend as much on the availability of the remedy itself as on the hazards of continued irradiation, and the circumstances of different accidents or environmental contaminations will vary so widely that it may be inappropriate to set universal levels."

In other words, any action values or levels for an emergency will depend on the nature of the accident, the control measures available, the number of people involved, the duration of the exposure, and the likelihood of any repetition of the incident

In summary, it would appear that, to be meaningful, any guidance recommendations must take into account many factors which include not only possible dietary and economic consequences of the control action, but also the feasibility of introducing environmental controls at the expense of persons and activities within the economy in no way responsible for the situation which is supposed to be corrected. It would also appear that intervention of authorities to counteract an environmental radiation condition after it has been created requires a set of decisions which justify numerical values higher than those designed to limit the initial release of radioactivity to the environment by a continuing industry in normal peacetime operations. Consequently, the basic approach is to evaluate the need to introduce public protection measures on the basis of all circumstances extant when an unusual situation arises. A primary consideration in reaching this viewpoint is that the value of such protective steps is not measured by some predetermined exposure which the public would be allowed to accept regardless of the cause. Rather, the value of such countermeasures is directly determined by the amount of exposure which is *not* received, in comparison with that which would be received if countermeasures were not undertaken. A fundamental requirement for a meaningful decision is prior knowledge as to how much exposure might reasonably be anticipated in the future if protective action is not taken, and the initiation of corrective actions at a low level if it is anticipated that such actions will be in the public interest.

The selection of any of these levels is, therefore, a matter of profound judgment since the important factors cannot be put into a mathematical equation that comes out with an answer labeled "a calculation of the benefit versus the risk."

THE U.S. ATOMIC ENERGY COMMISSION AND RADIOLOGICAL EMERGENCY ASSISTANCE

F. RAYMOND ZINTZ
U.S. Atomic Energy Commission
Washington, D.C.

A DISCUSSION of the U.S. Atomic Energy Commission and radiological emergency assistance might best begin with some background information as to why the U.S. Atomic Energy Commission supports a nation-wide program of radiological emergency assistance. First of all, it should be recognized that the Atomic Energy Commission has a general responsibility to protect the health and safety of the public while contributing to the development, use and control of nuclear energy under the provisions of the Atomic Energy Act of 1954 as amended. In Section 3 of the Act, Congress has stated its intention to provide for a widespread atomic energy program consistent with the health and safety of the public. With this in mind, it does not seem unusual that, throughout the history of the Atomic Energy Program, assistance has been given from time to time to those in need of help when they were involved with radiological safety problems. Some of these problems resulted from incidents with radioactive material.

The Atomic Energy Commission's radiological emergency assistance could be said to have started on an organized basis because of the need to be prepared for the possibility of accidents in nuclear weapons research, development, production and testing activities. In order to meet this need, the Atomic Energy Commission, in cooperation with the Department of Defense, established specially trained emergency teams. Also, the Atomic Energy Commission's Licensing and Regulation Program became active with the 1954 revision of the Atomic Energy Act. This program encouraged a steady growth in the number of private users of radioactive materials. The necessity to be prepared for radiation accidents involving hazards to the public health and safety became more apparent than ever from the experience in 1957 with the Kellogg Company incident in Texas, and the Windscale reactor accident in England.

These and some other factors influenced the decision of the General Manager of the Atomic Energy Commission to issue, in June of 1958, an Atomic Energy Commission Radiological Assistance Plan establishing the organization and procedures for coordinating the capability of the Atomic Energy Commission and the Department of Defense for handling radiological incidents. The Plan covers both weapon and non-weapon incidents arising in on-site contractor operations, off-site contractor or licensee establishments, and in other places as reported by military or civil authorities or others. It was made clear in the Plan that the assistance provided and the responsibility assigned in the Plan was not intended to abridge state and local authority in any way. Under this Plan, the United States is divided into eight geographical regions for radiological assistance. In each region, an Atomic Energy Commission office is assigned the responsibility for providing radiological assistance in emergencies involving radioactive material (Figure VII-1). In regional order, these eight are the New York, Oak Ridge, Savannah River, Albuquerque, Chicago, Idaho, San Francisco, and Richland Operations Offices. Note that the Virgin Islands and Puerto Rico are included in Region 2 under Oak Ridge, while the Canal Zone is included in Region 3 under Savannah River. Each of these offices maintains a radiological emergency response capability available upon request twenty-four hours a day.

In addition to its other responsibilities for radiological assistance in Region 4, the Albuquerque Operations Office is responsible for radiological emergency operating procedures and instructions pertaining to Atomic Energy Commission coordination and cooperation with the Department of Defense. This is accomplished through a Joint Nuclear Accident Coordinating Center, called JNACC, which is established in accordance with the provisions of a Joint Atomic Energy Commission–Department of Defense Agreement. This coordinating center is located at Sandia Base, Albuquerque, New Mexico, and is staffed by the Field Command Headquarters of the Defense Atomic Support Agency for the Department of Defense, and the Albuquerque Operations Office for the Atomic Energy Commission.

U.S. ATOMIC ENERGY COMMISSION

REGIONAL OFFICE AREAS
OF RESPONSIBILITY FOR
RADIOLOGICAL ASSISTANCE
IN INCIDENTS INVOLVING
RADIOACTIVE MATERIALS

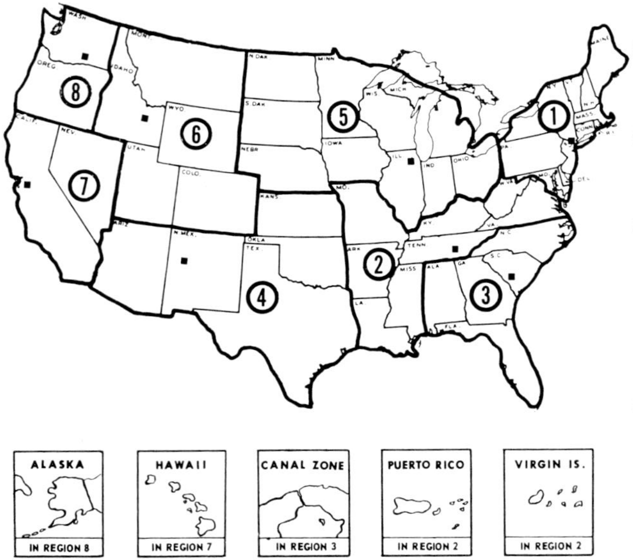

REGION NO. and OPERATIONS OFFICE	POST OFFICE ADDRESS	TELEPHONE for ASSISTANCE	DDD AREA CODE
1 NEW YORK	376 HUDSON STREET NEW YORK, NEW YORK 10014	YUKON 9-1000	212
2 OAK RIDGE	P. O. BOX E OAK RIDGE, TENNESSEE 37831	483-8611, Ext. 7607 or 483-7486	615
3 SAVANNAH RIVER	P. O. BOX A AIKEN, S.C. 29802	N. AUGUSTA, S.C. 824-6331, Ext. 3333 AIKEN, S. C. 649-6211, Ext. 3333	803
4 ALBUQUERQUE	P. O. BOX 5400 ALBUQUERQUE, NEW MEXICO 87115	264-4667	505
5 CHICAGO	9800 S. CASS AVE. ARGONNE, ILLINOIS 60439	739-7711 Ext. 2111 duty hrs. Ext. 4011 off hrs.	312
6 IDAHO	P. O. BOX 2108 IDAHO FALLS, IDAHO 83401	522-4400 Ext. 2345	208
7 SAN FRANCISCO	2111 BANCROFT WAY BERKELEY, CALIFORNIA 94704	THORNWALL 1-5620	415
8 RICHLAND	P. O. BOX 550 RICHLAND, WASHINGTON 99352	942-1111 Ext. 6-5441	509

Revised: September 1964

FIGURE VII-1. U.S. Atomic Energy Commission Radiological Assistance Regions and Emergency Telephone Numbers.

The Joint Atomic Energy Commission—Department of Defense Agreement provides for mutual assistance between the two agencies in any radiological emergency. In addition to the Atomic Energy Commission radiological assistance teams that can be dispatched from thirty-nine Atomic Energy Commission facilities, the military services have radiation emergency teams at more than 300 military installations throughout the United States and overseas. This combined capability provides extensive coverage for prompt response throughout the United States.

Although the resources of the Atomic Energy Commission and Department of Defense (Figure VII-2) are considerable, they will

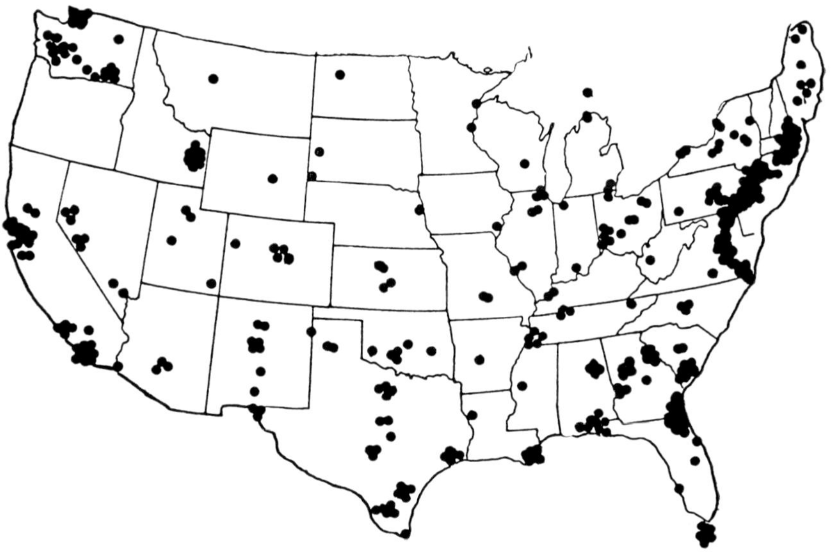

FIGURE VII-2. Distribution of Nuclear Accident Response Capabilities of the Department of Defense and the U.S. Atomic Energy Commission.

be supplemented with the additional resources of ten other Federal agencies which, in 1961, became signatories to an Interagency Radiological Assistance Plan. The Interagency Plan which is being put into effect provides for the integration of the participating agencies' capabilities to render advice and assistance in the event of radiation incidents. It also provides for the development of coordination with state and local health, police, fire and civil defense agencies and

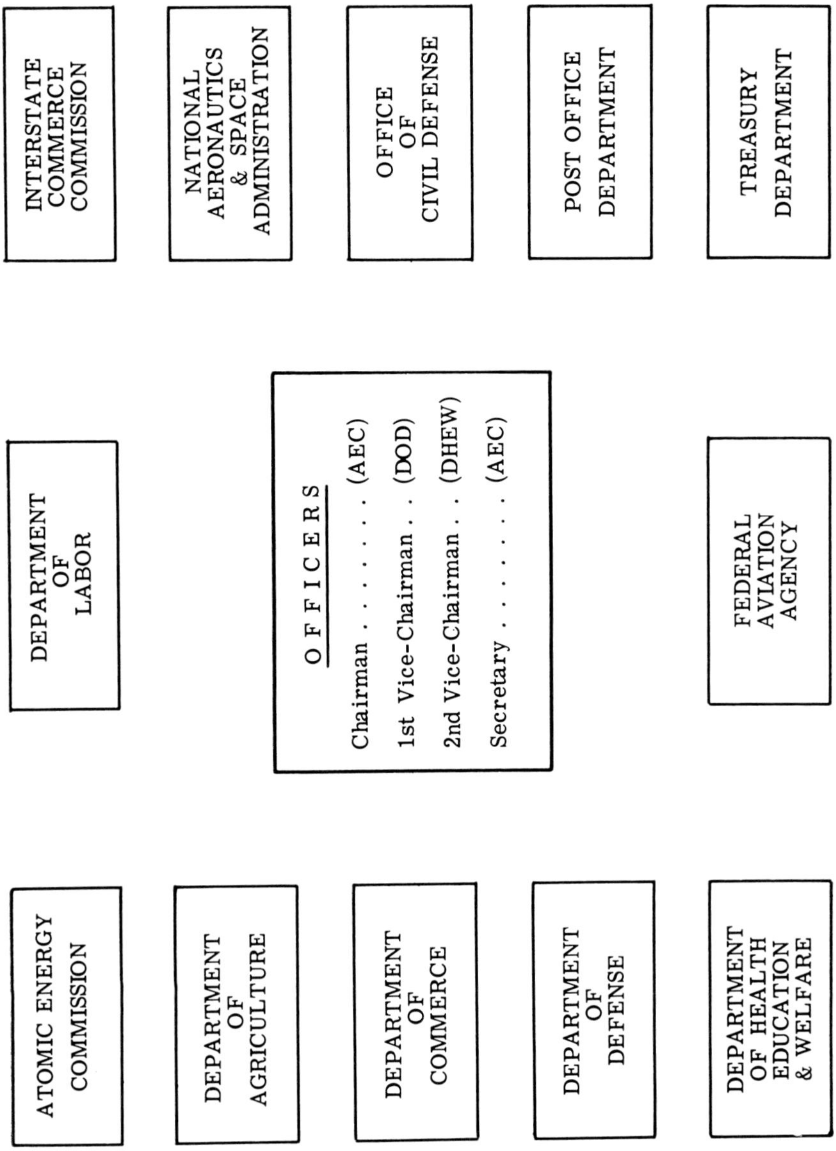

FIGURE VII-3. Interagency Committee on Radiological Assistance showing participating Agencies and Organization.

development of a radiological incident training program. This program is intended to provide instruction and a method of implementation for training personnel of federal, state and local agencies who may be expected to cope with incidents involving radioactive material. Under the Interagency Plan, the Atomic Energy Commission has primary responsibility for the administration and implementation of the Plan.

An Interagency Committee on Radiological Assistance (Figure VII-3), comprised of authorized representatives of each signatory agency, is provided by the Plan. This committee is responsible for obtaining the approval of the signatory agencies on the interpretation of policy and changes in the Interagency Plan; and for assuring the respective agencies that activities related to the implementation of the Plan will be consistent with the authority and responsibility contained in federal statutes and executive orders applicable to the participating federal agencies.

The provisions of the Interagency Plan are now in effect and guide the interagency relations of the federal agencies in radiological emergency arrangements for cooperation and coordination. As a contribution to the Interagency Plan training program, the Atomic Energy Commission has published a document prepared for the Interagency Committee on Radiological Assistance. Its title is *Radiological Emergency Procedures for the Non-Specialist.* This publication is designed to provide fundamental and reliable information which the ordinary layman can use for guidance in taking immediate action in case of accidents involving radioactive material. It is illustrated and can be used for talks to a lay audience. Copies are for sale by the Superintendent of Documents, U.S. Printing Office, Washington, D.C. (20402), at thirty-five cents a copy. Other Interagency Committee projects include a survey to identify the radiological emergency resources available from the twelve participating federal agencies and instructions as to the organization and the procedures by which to utilize these resources in radiological emergency operations. The resources information is so extensive that an automatic data processing system is being developed to handle it. It is hoped that the initial instructions and procedures approved by the Interagency Committee will be put into effect before the end of 1964. In the meantime, however, the capabilities of the Atomic Energy Commission, Department of Defense, U.S. Public Health Service, U.S. Coast Guard, and several other agencies are active in providing protection for the public health and safety from the results of incidents involving radioactive material.

Let us now turn again to the Atomic Energy Commission Radiological Assistance Program. This Program is based on a policy of making available from Atomic Energy Commission resources such radiological advice and assistance as may be appropriate to minimize injury to people, to minimize loss of property, to cope with radiological hazards, and to protect the public health and safety. Assistance is available upon request from Atomic Energy Commission contractors, licensees, federal, state and local agencies, private organizations, or individuals in the event of incidents believed to involve material defined, by the Atomic Energy Act of 1954 and amendments, as source, byproduct or special nuclear material, or material that may be obtained under a license issued by a state having an agreement with the Atomic Energy Commission, pursuant to Section 274b of the Atomic Energy Act, or ionizing radiation sources used in Atomic Energy Commission supported work. In other words, the Atomic Energy Commission, when asked for help by someone involved in an incident with radioactive materials, will provide such advice and assistance as it can to protect the public health and safety or the safety of individuals.

Since emergency assistance is necessarily something that must be available at any hour of any day, each of the eight regional offices has a special telephone number to receive requests for radiological emergency assistance. The type of assistance provided will depend considerably upon the immediate hazard to people, the kind and quantity of radioactive material involved, the location of the incident, and who is believed to be responsible for the radioactive material. It has often been possible to meet a request for assistance by giving the proper advice (see Appendix VII-1) or by requesting that the appropriate state, local or federal agency provide the necessary assistance. However, to the extent considered appropriate, Atomic Energy Commission radiological assistance may include radiological monitoring; emergency sampling and radiation monitoring of materials including air, food and water; radiological decontamination advice and emergency assistance; medical advice on the handling and treatment of people exposed to radiation or radioactive material; special laboratory services needed for the evaluation of personnel radiation exposure and environmental radiological hazards; and specialists in nuclear weapons accident operations. If the emergency situation warranted it, the Atomic Energy Commission, from its laboratories and production plants, could bring a considerable amount of additional resources to bear on the task of protecting health and safety.

In addition to the fixed facilities and the thousands of technically trained personnel employed there, equipment and material are available which could be used in off-site radiological emergency operations. Examples of some specialized U.S. Atomic Energy Commission equipment are the Oak Ridge National Laboratory Mobile Dosimetry Laboratory; the Sandia Corporation special fire-fighting truck to accompany and protect certain radioactive material when it is in transit; and portable aerial survey instrumentation which is used routinely for maintaining surveillance over environmental radiation levels both on-site and off-site at several Atomic Energy Commission installations. Of particular interest is an Aerial Radiological Monitoring System (ARMS) that is presently installed in a Beech Model 50 twin Bonanza aircraft. This system was developed under an Atomic Energy Commission Division of Biology and Medicine research and development contract. The primary objective is to develop an accurate, analytical, sensitive, rugged and compact radiological measurement system for aerial survey of natural background radiations and of levels higher than natural background. Background surveys of more than fifty geographical areas in the United States have been made to obtain the radiological information, as well as to test the system under operating conditions. Technical reports on the system have been published and are designated by the letters CEX followed by a number (i.e., CEX-59.4, CEX-60.3). The ARMS is available for Atomic Energy Commission emergency survey missions and is capable of outlining accurately an area contaminated with 1 μc of iodine-131 per square meter on the ground from an altitude of 500 feet.

When an Atomic Energy Commission team arrives at the scene of an incident it may, in general, do four things: 1) monitor for radiation to evaluate the hazard and determine the emergency measures needed to protect health and safety; 2) coordinate the emergency operations in cooperation with local authorities at the scene; 3) provide information for the public, and 4) provide emergency medical advice and, if necessary to save life or minimize injury, carry out emergency measures to assist people who may be injured as a result of the incident. However, when a more appropriate authority arrives at the scene, the Atomic Energy Commission team captain will relinquish control of the emergency operations to this authority.

When the emergency period is over, the person or agency responsible for the radioactive material, the site, or the facilities involved would be expected to provide for the necessary post-emergency decontamination and recovery operation, unless this responsibility has been accepted by someone else. Atomic Energy Commission radiological emergency assistance, however, would not be withdrawn from the scene until appropriate steps had been taken to give reasonable assurance that the public health and safety will be protected from any remaining potential hazards.

As might be expected, the incident experience has been quite diversified. The Atomic Energy Commission has responded to requests for assistance in incidents ranging from fake packages of radioactive materials to the actual contamination of buildings, public roads, railroads, and other property. Since there is not time to discuss these incidents in detail, perhaps a few statistics will give you some idea of the activity which has been experienced. During the period from July 1958 through December 1962, the Atomic Energy Commission responded to a total of 378 requests for radiological assistance (Figure VII-4), not including hundreds of requests for technical information, the loan of movie films, lecturers, copies of publications, and other help and advice. Among the 378 responses, assistance was sent to the scene in 182 incidents, but in 196 responses advice was adequate to assist the authorities at the scene. It is of interest to note that radioactive material was actually involved in 205 of the incidents and in 173, radioactive material was not involved. Although averages are relatively meaningless, this comes out to be an average of approximately seven responses per month for the total period. During 1963, the Atomic Energy Commission responded to 57 requests for radiological assistance. Assistance was sent to the scene in twenty-eight of these cases. Radioactivity was involved in forty-two of the fifty-seven incidents.

YEAR	TOTAL NUMBER OF REQUESTS	ASSISTANCE SENT TO SCENE	ADVICE ONLY*	RADIOACTIVE MATERIAL WAS INVOLVED	
				Yes	No
1958-59	92	67	25	42	50
1960	79	37	42	54	25
1961	139	41	98	58	81
1962	68	37	31	51	17
TOTALS	378	182	196	205	173

FIGURE VII-4. U.S. Atomic Energy Commission Radiological Assistance Responses for the period July 1958 through December 1962.*

From time to time, there has been an interest in knowing the percentage of responses made to different kinds or categories of incidents. In order to shed some light upon this, a study of 223 radiological assistance responses made during the years 1960, 1961 and 1962 was undertaken. The result showed that 40 per cent of the incidents involved transportation, 22 per cent were on site, 15 per cent were referred to other agencies for response, 10 per cent occurred off site, 10 per cent were due to pranks, and 3 per cent were related to reports of alleged radioactive fallout. During this three-year period and, in fact, from the beginning of the Atomic Energy Program, the Atomic Energy Commission has not had to deal with a radiation accident seriously affecting off-site areas. However, this shortage of serious accidents does not dull our efforts to be prepared. We shall continue to work on the implementation of the Interagency Plan. We shall offer more encouragement to state and local agencies to develop their emergency capabilities. We shall carry on the work toward improving the Atomic Energy Commission radiological assistance capabilities, and develop additional data and information which can be used in training and planning for emergency operations.

Appendix VII-1

AEC-Recommended Instructions for Immediate Emergency Action in Incidents Involving Radioactive Materials

When incidents involve a nuclear radiation source, the spillage or

*Even though radioactive material is involved, experience has shown that telephoned advice is often adequate to assist the authorities at the scene.

release of radioactive material, or there are personal injuries in incidents involving radioactive materials, the following emergency actions and precautions against radiation exposure should apply:

1) Notify immediately ....
at .... The telephone number is ....

2) If the incident involves wreckage and a person is believed to be alive and trapped, make every effort possible to rescue him.

3) Restrict the area involved as a result of the incident. Keep the public as far from the scene of the incident as practical. Souvenir collection and handling of debris by onlookers should be prevented.

4) Segregate and detain for further examination those persons who have had possible contact with the radioactive material. Obtain the names and addresses of those involved.

5) Remove injured persons from the area affected by the incident with as little direct personal contact as possible and hold them at a transfer point. Until physicians familiar with radiological health procedures are present, limit first aid and medical procedures to those that must be done promptly. Whenever recommended by a doctor, an injured individual should be removed to a hospital or office for treatment, and the doctor or hospital should be informed when there is reason to suspect that the injured individual may have radioactive contamination on his body or clothing.

6) In incidents involving fire, fight fires from upwind whenever possible. Treat as a fire involving toxic chemicals. Keep out of smoke, fumes, or dust resulting from the incident. Segregate clothing and tools used at the fire until they can be checked for radioactive contamination. Do not handle suspected material until it has been monitored and released by radiation-monitoring personnel.

7) In the event of a vehicle accident involving radioactive material, detour all traffic around the accident scene. If this is not possible, move the vehicle or vehicles involved the shortest distance necessary to clear the right of way. If radioactive material is spilled, prevent the passage of vehicles and people through the area unless absolutely necessary. If right of way must be cleared before the

radiological assistance team arrives, wash spillage to the shoulders of the right of way with a minimum dispersal of wash water.

8) DO NOT eat, drink, or smoke in the incident area. Do not use food or drinking water that may have been in contact with material from the incident area.

9) DO NOT try to do too much prior to the arrival of radiation protection specialists and physicians.

THE ROLE OF THE PUBLIC HEALTH SERVICE IN RADIATION EMERGENCIES

RAYMOND T. MOORE
Division of Radiological Health
U.S. Public Health Service
Department of Health, Education, and Welfare
Dallas, Texas

Due to legal and practical considerations, major responsibilities for public health protection of the population of the United States are vested in the various state governments, functioning through the state health departments.

Through tradition, and also under federal statutes and regulations, the principal role of the United States Public Health Service is to assist and advise the states, and to conduct or support research and training programs. However, the Public Health Service has certain direct protective health responsibilities, involving for the most part activities of an international, national, or interstate nature, such as foreign quarantine or the safety of food and water served for human consumption on interstate common carriers.

Nevertheless, the history of public health in this country is replete with instances where, in an emergency, the Public Health Service has acted in vigorous concert with one or more states to cope with particular problems. Similar cooperative efforts and programs have also been undertaken with other federal agencies to solve health-related problems arising from program responsibilities of these other agencies.

The characteristics of several of the sources of potentially hazardous radiation have required that, in the rapidly evolving Federal-State radiological health programs, all of the operating patterns mentioned above have become important segments of the program administered by the Division of Radiological Health of the Public Health Service.

Before I describe the Division's activities in detail, a brief review of some of the events leading up to its formation might be in order. One of the first organized efforts in the field of radiation by the Public

Health Service was an investigation, during the early 30's, of radium poisoning among clock and watch dial painters. This was followed in the 40's by studies of x-ray and radium hazards in hospitals; cooperation with the Manhattan District on formulation of standards of human tolerance to radiation; and investigations involving the biological effects of exposure in animals. These and other efforts led to the acceptance, in 1954, of responsibility by the Service for off-site monitoring in support of the weapons testing program at the Nevada Test Site and, subsequently, of similar responsibilities in connection with tests conducted in the Pacific. These programs, continued over the years, provided an opportunity to perfect monitoring skills and to train numerous federal and state public health personnel in these skills.

In 1958, national interest in the subject, together with the growth of Public Health Service activity in radiation protection, led to the formation of a Division of Radiological Health with the assigned mission of developing a comprehensive program, including strengthened capability within the states and communities.

As a result of increased supportive activity at the Nevada Test Site, the first Regional Radiological Health Laboratory was opened by the Division at Las Vegas, Nevada, in 1959. As further needs arose, additional laboratories were opened at Montgomery, Alabama, and Winchester, Massachusetts, as well as special-purpose laboratories at Cincinnati, Ohio, and Rockville, Maryland. The Public Health Service's nationwide radiation surveillance programs, which are operated in conjunction with state agencies, are dependent on these laboratories. In the event of a radiological accident or emergency, personnel and technical assistance are available—on call—to the respective state health departments that need them. Each laboratory is also a training center and has various roles in research.

I. Support to States

In each of the nine Public Health Service Regions, there is now a Program Director for Radiological Health. These men are well trained in radiation per se, as well as in the health aspects of radiation. Because of their intimate knowledge of the states and their problems, they are key personnel for consultation, advice, and regional coordination.

A. ***Assignment of Personnel.*** At the present time, there are some 38 federal officers assigned to the states. These men occupy responsible positions in the state health departments and, in many instances, have furnished a nucleus for a state in building its own radiological health programs. While these officers are working in the individual states, they are under the control of, and responsible to, the state health officer.

B. ***Formula Grants Program.*** By the end of fiscal year 1963, all fifty states, plus Puerto Rico and the Virgin Islands, were participating in this program. The program makes money available to the states on a formula basis that takes into account the relative need for radiological health activities. The matching is done by a one-to-one formula. This money may be used for training, for personnel, or for equipment. Thus, each state does have a radiological health program. The activities vary with the anticipated needs and the resources available. However, each state can now provide some assistance in alleviating or controlling any radiation emergency which may occur within its boundaries.

II. Training

It is not easy to prepare for an accident or emergency when the exact location, magnitude, and probable effects are unknown. The Public Health Service has felt that this problem could be attacked by creating as large a pool of trained people as budget and personnel would allow. Thus, our training effort has largely been channeled along the following avenues:

Intramural. For many years, the Public Health Service has been conducting short courses (three weeks or less) in radiological health. These courses are conducted by Public Health Service personnel and are designed for employees of state and local health departments, as well as for Public Health Service personnel who need training in radiological health. During the fiscal year 1964, some fifty-two separate sessions have been scheduled, with a total of eighty-three or more weeks of training. In the main, this aspect of the training program is geared to meet the needs of state and local health departments.

Extramural or Outside of Service. Every year, a certain number of Public Health Service Officers are sponsored to attend the graduate schools of major United States universities. These assignments are usually made for one year and are designed to meet a specific Service need. A total of seventy-six Public Health Service personnel were supported in long-term "Outside the Service" graduate training in radiological health for the fiscal years 1960-62.

Training Grants to Universities. Training grants to universities to improve, expand, or establish radiation health specialist criteria were made available for the first time in the fiscal year 1961 by the Congress. Some fifteen universities then received grants for staff, equipment, or student assistance. As of July 1, 1963, there were twenty-eight major universities participating in this program.

Bench Training. This aspect of training cannot be overlooked. Bench-type trainees spend a variable length of time at one of our laboratories in order to master some particular technique.

III. Medical Liaison Officer Network

As a means of assisting the Atomic Energy Commission in investigating claims of radiobiological injury, a Medical Liaison Officer Network has been established by the Public Health Service. This is a network composed of physicians, usually on the staffs of the State Departments of Health, who are available for rapid investigation of situations in which a question has arisen as to whether or not an illness or disability may be due to the activities of the weapons testing or Plowshare programs. In this type of investigation, emphasis is placed on early determination of the individual's physical condition. Thus, the opinion of an individual's personal physician becomes extremely important. If there is, in fact, demonstrable injury, the State Health Officer, the Public Health Service, as well as the Atomic Energy Commission need to be made aware of this fact immediately.

IV. Interagency Plans

The *Interagency Radiological Assistance Plan,* published by the Department of Health, Education, and Welfare in July, 1961, defines responsibilities of signatory agencies concerning assistance to state and local authorities in handling radiological incidents.

In addition, we have a specific agreement with the United States Air Force to cover incidents involving certain nuclear materials. Definite procedures have been established for dealing with such incidents. If the Public Health Service is called upon, its immediate concern is to provide the assistance necessary to evaluate the hazard, counteract and control any acute danger, and to assist local and state health authorities and the Air Force as necessary. This may include the dispatch of Public Health Service radiological assistance teams. If such be the case, the functions of these teams may include:

A) Evaluation of the immediate radiation hazard.

B) Control of radiation sources to minimize the spread of radioactive contaminations.

C) Recommending action to minimize radiation exposure and property damage.

D) Examination of potentially exposed people and their food, air, and water supplies.

E) Reporting findings to the Air Force and the state health agency concerned.

Each team maintains its emergency monitoring kit on a "ready-for-use" basis.

Upon arrival at the scene, the Public Health Service emergency team works with Air Force and local health authorities. The teams are expected to take such action to protect life and property as will be consistent with the direction of local authority at the incident site.

Radium accidents, including lost or leaking sources, continue to be the most prevalent of radiation incidents. The Public Health Service has intensified its efforts in the area of radium control. To assist state health departments in planning programs for control of radium, the State Assistance Branch has distributed an evaluation of radium management information, a comprehensive bibliography on radium, an incident report sheet, a bibliography and outline of leak-testing procedures, and information on the location and quantity of radium in the various states.

To illustrate how the general build-up of radiological health in a state contributes to its overall accident competence, let us consider a situation which occurred recently.

There was a large explosion at a military base in one of our bigger states. The facts as known immediately were—"There was a large explosion at a secret base on the outskirts of a city. There was a mushroom cloud and windows were broken fifteen miles away." With only this amount of information, the state had activated its emergency plan; had ascertained the direction of the wind; had dispatched properly equipped monitors into the area; and had located high-volume air samplers in the projected path of the fallout, should there be any. The state plan also allowed for other units of the state government to provide for crowd control, public health, etc. (The explosion was of chemical origin, fortunately.)

As the volume of radiation users and usages increases, there is also an increasing likelihood of radiation incidents or emergencies. These will occur largely within areas where an individual state has primary responsibility for civilian health. Thus, our best approach to radiation accident control is through increased competence in radiological health in state and local health departments, as well as in the academic and civilian communities. To that end we have channeled the bulk of our efforts.

THE ROLE OF THE STATE IN LOCAL RADIATION EMERGENCIES

LYLE D. THOMAS
Division of Radiological Health
U.S. Public Health Service
Chicago, Illinois

STATE AND LOCAL health authorities have the prime responsibility for health protection of population groups within their jurisdiction. Radioactive material is just one of many contaminants introduced into man's environment for which control must be provided to protect the health and safety of the people. With the development and growth of state radiological health programs in recent years, these agencies are taking a more active role in meeting their responsibilities in the event of local radiation accidents and emergencies.

The history of radiological health is somewhat unique in that a federal agency was and is charged with the health and safety considerations by means of a regulatory program for reactor-produced radioisotopes and certain other radioactive materials. Wartime, and the "cloak of secrecy" associated with the applications of radioactive materials, played a major role in determining the level of administration; but the lack of competent personnel in this new and highly technical field at the state level was equally important. This picture is changing now as more and more states are acquiring highly trained technical personnel and developing comprehensive radiological health programs. The tooling and planning to cope with radiation emergencies are being integrated into the overall program at the state level.

Most states now have enabling legislation and specific regulations for radiation protection. In Region V of the Public Health Service, which includes the states of Illinois, Indiana, Michigan, Ohio, and Wisconsin, four of the five states have specific radiation legislation which includes authorizing the Governor to enter into an agreement with the U.S. Atomic Energy Commission for assumption of regulatory control over certain radioactive materials. In the state which lacks such enabling legislation at this time, there are regulations pertaining to the control of ionizing radiation. Thus, the basic authority exists.

Paralleling the development of state radiological health programs, currently over half of the states in the United States provide emergency team assistance and about one third provide orientation training to ancillary personnel such as police and firemen.

State radiological health programs include resources applicable to the handling of local radiation emergencies, namely: 1) a trained radiological health staff; 2) adequate instrumentation; and 3) a comprehensive communications network. These resources can be coordinated to provide emergency team assistance when requested, or to take action to protect the public health when needed.

Trained personnel is a "must" for conducting a state radiological health program. The same personnel provides the core of the capability for handling radiation emergencies. These persons are normally located centrally within the state, so that expert assistance is available within only a matter of a few hours at most from the scene of an emergency. Prior arrangements can and should be made to utilize local expertise upon request where it exists, e.g., in universities and local health agencies.

The basic instrumentation needed for most emergencies is already available and maintained in operating condition for routine radiological health program use. Consideration must be given to providing adequate back-up instrumentation for emergency purposes. Other miscellaneous supplies needed primarily for emergencies should be maintained in one or more readily available kits. Such supplies should include protective clothing for personnel, respirators, personnel dosimetry devices (dosimeters and film badges), air samplers, solid and liquid sample containers, decontamination kits, rope, portable lights, etc. Routine procedures should be established for periodically checking and exchanging batteries needed for all of this equipment. An operations manual prescribing basic procedures, possibly supplemented with check lists, should also be contained within the kit. All personnel subject to call for emergency monitoring duty should be intimately familiar with the instrumentation and the content of the kits.

An effective communications network must be established to expedite the services required to handle a radiation emergency. The communications channels for the reporting of radiation incidents are established by federal as well as state regulations for licensees of radiation sources. Even here, periodic visits to the radiation installations by representatives of the responsible state agency are needed to reinforce this working relationship.

The emergencies that can and do occur en route within our transportation systems necessitate broader planning and more elaborate preparation by the responsible state agencies. The state police are normally the first officials at the scene of an accident; they are equipped with a communications network reaching all corners of the state. This provides health officials with immediate notification of incidents, and establishes a direct communication line to the scene for gathering additional information helpful in ascertaining the type and scope of resources needed to cope with a given incident. The operations office of the state police should be supplied with the names and telephone numbers, in proper order, of individuals to contact in an emergency, and with copies of a questionnaire to complete, requesting basic information relevant to the incident.

In order to realize fully the resources available through the state police, a basic radiological training program should be initiated. To provide immediate information that radioactive materials are involved in an accident, it may be necessary to require knowledge of U.S. Interstate Commerce Commission labeling practices, or familiarization with the manner in which shipments of radioactive materials are listed in bills of lading. Initial assessment by state police officers of potential radiation exposure of individuals in the immediate area can be accomplished with very basic instrumentation and with a minimum of training. Such instrumentation may be available through Office of Civil Defense channels as a part of its endeavor to establish a statewide emergency monitoring capability. The training of state police personnel and the establishing of operational guidelines should be accomplished by the state radiological health staff. Action initiated by trained state police officers prior to the arrival of a radiological emergency team could very well transform a potential tragedy into a minor accident.

In most states, the most expeditious form of transportation of team personnel and their equipment to the site would be the automobile. Prior arrangements should be negotiated with the state police agency for providing transportation in those cases where expediency would thus be achieved.

During a three-year assignment with the Indiana State Board of Health, I had the opportunity to participate in the development of a radiological health program. Developing a comprehensive plan for handling radiation emergencies involves much planning, training, coordinating, and then revising as dictated by experience. Indiana has experienced nineteen known radiation incidents since 1958, ranging from very minor ones, resulting in no public health hazard, to incidents involving excessive exposure* to individuals as calculated from known parameters. The sources of radiation which were involved included radium, strontium, cobalt, tritium, krypton, iodine, uranium, x-radiation and others. Some of these emergency situations resulted from highway accidents, others from leaking sealed sources, and yet others from unjustified misuse. Although most of these incidents were not of a serious nature, all of them pointed clearly to the need for a well-organized plan and provided valuable experience toward its achievement. Indiana's plan follows essentially the pattern discussed in this paper.

Incidents involving radioactive materials have occurred in the past and will undoubtedly increase in number in future years. Many states now have workable plans, and other states are actively engaged in developing them. Even though federal emergency teams are available to provide required assistance, the states are not accepting this as relieving them of their basic responsibility in this field. The role of the state in local radiation emergencies is firmly established.

DISCUSSION

Dr. L. H. Lanzl: I should like to ask Mr. Zintz a hypothetical question. Suppose a private hospital had a radioactive spill. There is certain information which I think would be valuable. Would there be any cost to that hospital if it called you in and you came and offered some advice, or if the Atomic Energy Commission did some decontaminating? In addition, how does this overlap the work of private concerns which operate in this area?

*In excess of 3 rem to the whole body or one or more of the critical organs, within a calendar quarter.

Mr. F. R. Zintz: I think it is appropriate for Mr. William Brobst (U.S. Atomic Energy Commission, Chicago Operations Office, Health and Safety Division) to answer that.

Mr. W. A. Brobst: Sometimes the people who call us are a bit frightened at calling upon a government agency for help. We use a rather simple approach in Chicago. We will help anybody who calls, or we will make sure that they get help. If this involves sending a team from Argonne, we will send a team from Argonne, and ask questions later as to who is going to pay for this. Generally, we have taken care of the cost of emergency help ourselves. If somebody needs help, we will give help.

As far as decontamination efforts go, of course, this is up to the party responsible for the radioactive material. The radiological assistance plan is set up to provide emergency help by aiding in intelligently controlling the accident environs to prevent the spread of radioactive substances and minimizing harm to people or property.

As Mr. Zintz pointed out, most of the accidents which we have handled to date have been small. We send out people who will give advice and reassurance. If there is radioactivity involved, we give substantial, expert help. Generally speaking, we don't distinguish in Chicago between radium incidents and atomic-energy incidents. We answer any call we get as quickly as we can, and do not worry who will pay for it. The aim is to protect people and property.

Mr. F. L. Bordell (Westinghouse Atomic Power): Are there any plans between the governments of Mexico, the United States and Canada in the event there should be an incident where one government will call on a radiological assistance team of the other if need be?

Mr. F. R. Zintz: A short answer: no.

Dr. R. T. Moore: May I comment? I agree with his answer. However, our service has established liaison with the proper Canadian authorities as well as the proper authorities in Mexico. I would not want to say any more than that at the moment. I don't think the answer is an unqualified "no."

Mr. F. R. Zintz: I took it for granted that it is known that the Atomic Energy Commission has a liaison office in Chalk River, Canada, and that problems have been handled through this office. When asked if we have formal plans—I must answer, no.

Chairman R. K. Clark: It always seems to be important to distinguish between informal relations and formal ones. Often the informal relations turn out to be more effective.

Mr. W. B. Rivkin: My question is to Dr. Moore. He referred to assistance teams. Are these teams organized by the states? If they are state-organized, could we have some idea as to how many states have such teams; and are there other teams?

Dr. R. T. Moore: I was not referring at all to state-organized teams. I was referring to U.S. Public Health Service teams from the Division of Radiological Health. We do have quite a number of teams. There is one in each of our laboratories, ready to go. We have other trained people who can make up a second or third or fourth team, if needed.

Mr. R. G. Gallaghar: Some of the states have emergency monitoring teams. For example, in the Commonwealth of Pennsylvania, we are fortunate to have an emergency team. Some of the states are developing this capability within their own health departments.

Mr. F. R. Zintz: According to a recent questionnaire, if every state does as it says it is going to do, there will be on the order of thirty-two states in the future which will have emergency teams.

Mr. A. A. Weintraub: Dr. Moore, in the medical liaison officer network, are their investigations restricted solely to accidents that involve weapons and Plowshare?

Dr. R. T. Moore: Generally speaking, yes, although the capability could be used for other purposes.

Mr. A. A. Weintraub: It *could* be available for others?

Dr. R. T. Moore: It could be available for others. There would have to be a different agreement arranged, but it could be done.

Chapter VIII

THE ETHICAL PROBLEM

INTRODUCTORY REMARKS

LAWRENCE H. LANZL

Argonne Cancer Research Hospital
and Department of Radiology
The University of Chicago
Chicago, Illinois

THE DIVERSE ASPECTS of radiation accidents and emergencies which have been presented here dealt with the practical side of the problem. They included physical, biological, and medical sciences as well as public relations, psychological, and legal considerations. In conclusion, the moral and ethical aspects will be considered as well.

It has often been said that World War II was the physicists' war, since it was during this period that certain branches of physics, or at least their applications, developed and moved forward at a greatly accelerated pace. The consequences of these developments, particularly of the use of atomic energy in weapons, stirred the conscience of men even before the atomic bomb was used in combat. This initial concern was, of course, confined to the scientists working within the Manhattan Project. Since the war, the worldwide knowledge of the existence of atomic weapons has led to much debate on the morality of some scientific work. A demand for open discussion has been made by scientists as well as by the general public. Even among many of those persons who formerly considered science, both pure and applied, as the "be-all" and the "end-all" of life no longer considered this their position.

The moral problems related to the use of atomic energy and its ionizing radiations are much more complex than, say, those inherent in the use of the automobile. Through the development of the automobile, most of the human race has derived much pleasure as well as faster and more comfortable transportation. But cars have also given our metropolitan areas a severe traffic problem. In addition, they have given us tremendous annual death rates and even higher numbers of painful injuries. Yet the use of the automobile in itself causes no long-range genetic damage to the animal or plant kingdoms. (We are disregarding effects of hydrocarbons in automobile exhaust, and byproducts of wear of tires and roads.)

Ionizing radiations, however, have the demonstrated ability to cause somatic-cell as well as reproductive-cell damage. Thus, it is conceivable that the whole gene pool of humanity could be harmed if the effect of ionizing radiations became sufficiently widespread.

Here, we have been dealing only with the peacetime uses of radiation, such as the use of x-rays in medicine, of isotopes and accelerators in research and industry, and of the nuclear reactor for running ships, providing electrical power, or treating patients with brain tumors. The radiation due to these uses is added to the existing background.

When a radiation accident occurs in which living matter and particularly human beings receive a still higher radiation dose, the threat of increased genetic damage tends to emphasize the importance of considering the moral issue of the use of radiation. There may be those who believe that this matter can await the acquisition of more complete scientific knowledge on the extent of genetic damage; however, there may not be time—the damage may have been done.

In one sense, the problem confronting us is not a new one. We have seen in the past, for example, conservationists struggling against the onslaughts of industrialization and mechanized farming, to the extent that only a small percentage of land is now left untouched in this country. In this instance, we have the problem of human conservation from possible genetic damage, and from the thwarting of positive evolution.

The concluding essay by Dr. John H. Rust then, will be directed toward an answer to the moral and ethical questions raised by the peaceful use of atomic energy. Dr. Rust has had a distinguished career in several fields, as a veterinarian and veterinary pathologist, in biophysics, physiology, and pharmacology. In the last few years, he has devoted himself to the study of the implications of radiation for society. This work included a conference on radiation and social ethics.

Participants in this conference included leading theologians representing and, in some cases, speaking for the main world religions, as well as authorities in physics, medicine, genetics, biophysics, and other branches of science and the social sciences. With these studies as a background, Dr. Rust prepared the following paper.

IMPLICATIONS OF RADIATION FOR SOCIETY

JOHN H. RUST

Section of Nuclear Medicine
The University of Chicago
Chicago, Illinois

On several occasions I have said, and I know that others have thought so as well, that the advent of nuclear energy in the affairs of man was like opening Pandora's box. If you will recall, Pandora was the mythical woman who was the possessor of a box in which there was an evil spirit. When the box was opened against her advice and wishes, the evil spirit escaped and created havoc all over the world. Most of us who have heard this little story believe that it ends there; but there is one bit more to add. Something remained in the box. It was *hope.*

I will discuss the limitations on the *hope* expressed in the little story I have just mentioned in *the peaceful uses of nuclear energy.* At first one might believe that there is no problem. By definition, any peaceful uses of nuclear energy are, *a priori,* good. But it is not necessarily true. There are complex social consequences.

Nuclear science can serve as a prototype for all science. It is a problem of the moment, and all of us understand that to a substantial degree. You have heard some equate nuclear science with the invention of gun power, the bow and arrow, or the wheel. All had a profound impact upon the contemporary society and all were ambiguous, i.e., they could be used for both war and peace. In fact, there are few developments by man of a scientific or technical nature that don't have some ambiguity. It can be pointed out that the release of radioactive elements into man's environment creates somatic and particularly genetic mutations. Even in the peaceful uses of nuclear energy this is true. We are, therefore, polluting the gene pool; and those who share in that pool many generations hence will suffer for the acts of our time. However, it is overlooked that the invention of the steam engine also had ambiguous results. It is true that man did increase his control over his environment. In addition, he began to pollute his environment with noxious gases and debris which have cost the lives of many. His potential for waging destructive war was immeasurably increased. Many believe that he established a new and often a less desirable social order. This new, less desirable social order was that of grinding poverty and reduced human dignity which has been transmitted from generation to generaiton just as surely as though it were a dominant genetic inheritance. This I think of as a social inheritance, and I believe that it can be just as burdensome as deleterious genetic inheritance in the affairs of man. I give this example to define what I mean when I say that I believe scientific and technical development is not good in itself. It is only good if wisely used.

The basic problem, then, is the wise utilization of scientific information and of the technical developments which arise from it. Perhaps we should set up definitions. Scientific research is the search for truth in nature. Technology, which is often confused with scientific endeavors, is the application and utilization of the fruits of scientific research, i.e., scientific information. I make the distinction because there should be a deep and fundamental difference in the attitude toward them by society.

Scientific research, the search for truth in nature, must be unfettered. There are no theological arguments; no moralistic or other arguments that can deny this. The search for truth, whether it be by science, by poetry, by music, or whatever, is a noble pursuit in itself. The unraveling of the mysteries of nature is something like a religious experience and may well be akin to it. We are not surprised that those civilizations which restrict the scientist in his search also restrict the artist, the musician, and the scholar. It is a depression of the human spirit and a hurt to the dignity of all men when this occurs.

There is a rational excuse for the control of technology. No one can justly say that, because a cordwainer makes the best rope, he is to blame for the men hung by it. Is the botanist-scientist to blame for his effort to understand the Agave plant from which the sisal was derived to make the rope? Neither can he be blamed for the scientific truths and the technical developments, for they are ambiguous in their possible applications. Of course, where an evil end is known and is clearly dominant, a scientist or technologist can refuse to participate, or try to channel his work to good ends. But it is not easy to recognize such ends, and often this is a dilemma which cannot be resolved.

What is needed is an ethic for society. A theologically derived ethic for the individual is old and usually quite successful, but for society it is of modern origin and has not, as a rule, been very successful. St. Thomas Aquinas did not even seem to be interested in the problem. At least he does not mention it. To develop a social ethic adequate for our scientific and technical development, all members of the society should participate in the discussions and dialogues that shape it. The citizens must learn much more about the scientific method and about science and technology. Decisions made on the basis of half-understood truths are often worse than no decision at all. Scientists and technologists must participate in the teaching of the uninformed citizens, and they must participate in the dialogues that ensue. They must never dominate either the teaching or the dialogue. The shape of the social ethic must be fashioned in the interests of all citizens. It is to be remembered that a social ethic is derived from all human experience and reason—not just from the experience of the scientist or technologist.

The social, political, and economic actions of man are rarely in themselves completely good or completely evil, but contain some elements of both. Theologians call this the Principle of the Double Effect. Understanding this principle helps to establish an ethic for a social action that produces multiple effects, some good and some evil. We can consider the peaceful use of nuclear energy in this context and set up three guides that bear upon the matter. They are:

a) The use of nuclear energy should always be put to a morally good purpose.

b) The good that arises must be as a direct use of nuclear energy. An evil done to initiate a morally good end is not acceptable.

c) The good derived must outweigh the evil produced. Whether the evil be at the time of the good effect or even remote in time from it has no bearing upon the restriction.

It will be well to examine a few of the problems that arise from the peaceful uses of nuclear energy. I have already spoken of the ambiguity which arises from the utilization of scientific information. This is also true of nuclear energy. There can be few who will suggest that the purpose of using nuclear energy for the production of power is an evil one. In fact, most will admit that this is a morally good purpose. There is no obvious evil step on the way to the morally good end. Some might argue that the radioactive waste that is the end product of power production is potentially an evil because it can produce somatic and genetic injury in man. But this has not been to date an actual injury, nor does it have much of a potential for future injury since we have been, with rare exceptions, able to isolate all such wastes from man's environment. It is likely that this will remain so for any reasonably foreseeable future.

From this analysis, then, one must conclude that nuclear energy for power is morally good. Here there is little or no ambiguity. An ambiguity arises when one adds the sentence, "The power so derived will be used to produce instruments of war." It is further complicated when one qualifies the war by labeling it a "just" war. I suspect that the dilemma can be reduced to a meaningless level if one concludes that power from nuclear energy is not unique and, therefore, does not in itself become morally evil.

Another case is the failure to use nuclear energy for human needs. Arguments can be raised that nuclear energy produces no death-dealing fumes and fogs such as arise from fossil fuels and that, therefore, it is morally good, and that it is evil not to use it. Or, in certain countries with limited fuel resources, energy is needed also for the production of food, clothing, and medicine for the preservation of life. If these are not provided, freedom will be lost to authoritarian governments. Increased tensions will create dangers of international misunderstanding, and eventually wars. Here, then, one can say that power from nuclear energy is morally good, and that not to use it is evil. Without question, the use of nuclear energy for power in these cases answers positively each of the three caveats raised by the Principle of the Double Effect.

One of the most depressing cases is that of the disparity between the technologically developed and the developing nations. Nuclear science has put a premium upon persons of technical skill. In fact, it has created such a need that many more persons are attracted to technology than ever before. Frequently, some of the few who do exist in the developing nations are attracted to and stay permanently in the technologically developed nations. The technological gap tends to widen and the disparity between nations increases, until serious world tensions and unrest arise. This also happens within nations where the populations are not technologically homogeneous. In these instances, can one say that nuclear science is being put to a morally good purpose? The answer is probably yes. And if one is asked whether there is an evil done to achieve the morally good end, it is likely that one would not be able to deny it. Similarly, there may be a question about the good outweighing the evil. What can be done? The obvious answer is to close as quickly as possible the technological gap that exists between countries and between peoples within a country. There must be a sharing of the fruits of scientific and technological development between all men and all nations.

These examples are sufficient to demonstrate that the advent of nuclear energy in its peaceful applications brought its own special problems and intensified many others. They also tend to demonstrate that men of good will can reduce these problems to acceptable levels. It will take the active participation of us all. We must remember the hope that still remains.

NAME INDEX

SUBJECT INDEX

C

D

E

F

G

H

I

J

L

M

S